Hollywood Abbs
Without The Gym

Ilya Sulima

www.IlyaSulima.com

Photographer, Editor and Author: **Ilya Sulima**

www.ilyasulima.com

<u>Model name:</u> **Timothy Valencia**

www.facebook.com/TimVFit

<u>Model name:</u> **Derek Trudeau**

www.trudeaufitness.com

www.djtrudeau.com

<u>Model name:</u> **Brittni Johnson**

www.facebook.com/brittnij

ISBN: 978-0615749631
ISBN-13:0615749631

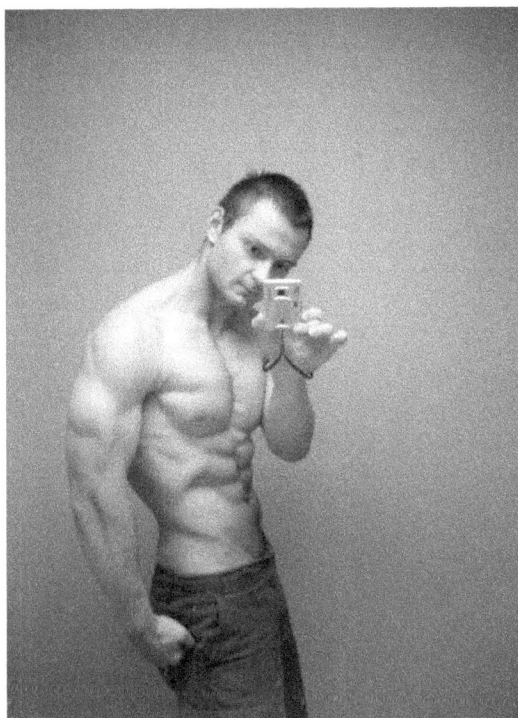

Ilya Sulima

To quote Sylvester from Rocky Balboa

" It ain't about how hard you hit, it's about how hard you can get hit and keep moving forward. It's about how much you can take and keep moving forward. That's how winning is done! Now if you know what you're worth then go out and get what you're worth but you gotta be willing to take the hit."

CHAPTER 1
THE OVERVIEW

The film stuck Hollywood abbs, do you have them?

A very crucial point to mention right off the bat is that many Hollywood stars who get in shape don't do it by themselves. They rely on professional help to get to a specific goal by a set deadline. Some stars even crash diet and train ridiculously hard to get those abbs out. The difference between the regular Joe and a Hollywood star is that the star is on a deadline and has no choice but to get in shape. The job is on the line. The regular Joe on the other hand may want to get those abbs out, but lacks the necessary motivation and perhaps a deadline. Unlike Joe, the movie star crosses to the enemy shores with his army and burns the ships so that retreat would not be an option.

It takes determination, cardio, resistance training and diet to get those abbs. Some stars even have two or three personal trainers that they work with. If you ever have the opportunity to observe a movie star train for a role, you will understand that it's a **full time job. I'm letting you know this so that there are no surprises as to why so many people fail to achieve that ripped fit Hollywood abbs look.**

Another very significant factor is food. Quite often the stars have their own personal chefs. These chefs are masters of cooking delicious dietary foods. Eating clean is more than half the battle. The average Joe may understand the basic concept of eating clean, but actually doing it is a whole different story. However, you unquestionably need not be discouraged. If you decide to focus on those abbs daily, with time you'll earn them.

(**Note**) Next time you're in the gym, have a look around. Do you see anyone going from one exercise to the other and literally not taking a break? Maybe you will find one person out of a thousand who trains at that intensity level, but for the most part everyone sticks to the basics. The basics alone will not cut it if you want those Hollywood abbs.

(**Note**) Protein shakes and more protein shakes is the name of the game for some stars. These low calorie, low carb, high protein muscle feeding drinks may not taste pleasant, but they certainly do the job.

(**Note**) Cardio, cardio and more cardio. The average Joe is defeated by the overwhelming boredom of the treadmill or the Stairmaster. The movie star in training for a film only wishes he or she can experience that boredom. The movie star isn't bored. The movie star is covered in sweat that drips down into a salty pool beneath. The legs are burning, the heart is racing, the whole body is shaking, and a feeling of weakness is coming on. Pushing oneself that hard is what it takes to get those abbs. The Joe would not be bored if he too pushed himself that hard.

The Levels of Progression

You can look at getting in shape in terms of 4 levels.

Level 1

- Working out for health

Level one is the standard workout approach a beginner might consider. At level 1, the individual frequents the gym 2 to 3 times per week without a set schedule. The average person at this level doesn't get the ripped Hollywood abbs look. However, he or she can benefit considerably in terms of general health. Simple weight resistance, cardiovascular training and an effort to select healthy foods may:

- Help fight stress

- Fight muscle loss

- Improve over all range of motion

- Generally aids with physical and mental longevity.

Level 2

- Working out for health and weight loss or weight maintenance.

The typical approach to level 2 is a dedicated workout schedule of 3 to 4 times per week. The individual makes an effort to eat clean foods but does not sacrifice the social life. Some weight loss may happen in level 2 because the weekly caloric intake is lowered. The weight loss is usually slow. Sometimes no significant weight loss happens at all, but a constant weight is maintained. Over all level 2 is a good moderate approach toward a healthy lifestyle.

Level 3

- Training for a toned body

The typical approach to level 3 is a dedicated training schedule of 4 to 6 times per week. Most people in level 3 take training very seriously and look at it as a lifestyle. These individuals make the time every week to get their workouts in. Most junk food, alcohol and "unhealthy fatty social events" are tackled with moderation or avoidance. Those who maintain a level 3 approach look significantly better than the average person. The problem some people face in level 3 is the yo-yo trap. Basically working out hard and then downright blowing the diet.

Level 4

- Training to look like a model and getting the abbs to show. This is the level at which the movie star trains when he or she is on a deadline to get that ripped Hollywood abbs look.

Some major factors in level 4 are:

- Caloric deficit through strict diet.

- Rigorous daily training 6-7 times per week. In extreme cases 2-3 times per day.

- Daily cardiovascular training of 1-3 hours.

- Large consumption of water, salads and lean meats.

- Supplement aids: Protein, amino acids, fat burners, fish oil, multivitamins etc…

Dangers of level 4 training if executed improperly

- Low blood sugar (weak overall feeling)

- Muscle strains

- Injury through ballistic training

- Over taxation of the adrenal gland through stimulants

- Loss of lean muscle tissue

The dangers may be avoided if the training approach is not constrained to tight time parameters. Instead of crashing to a goal in 3 short months, same results may be achieved in 6 months with wiggle room and avoidance of the danger factors.

Q and A

Should I jump into level 4 training right away?

NO. It's necessary to work your way up if you are not ready. Reading a book like Russian Ripped can guide you through the basics and get you up to speed.

What if I'm ready now?

If you are ready now because of an established training foundation then start taking names and kicking ass!

Should I have a physical and clearance before starting a training program from this book?

It is highly recommended that you have a thorough physical and clearance from your doctor before you start any training program including the one from this book.

Are supplements like fat burners dangerous?

Everyone reacts differently to fat burners and other supplementation. Rule of thumb is to focus on the diet first and never abuse any supplements if they are incorporated into the training program. However, there are many helpful high quality supplement aids on the market.

How long will it take for me to get my abbs out?

Every individual is different. Good looking abdominals are not magically given through miracles. They are earned through hard work. Some have more work than others. Be patient.

What will I need to do before I start a training program from this book?

- Read this book.

- Running shoes.

- Two moderate or light weight dumbbells.

- An mp3 player helps but it's not necessary.

What should I avoid?

- Junk food. A little bit of junk food every day keeps the abbs away but not the fat.

- Sodas.

- Negative influences. People who drag you down.

- Eating heavy meals before bed time.

- Excessive time spent on sedentary activities like television and video games.

- Giving supplementation priority over food. Food always comes first.

- Skipping meals.

- Habitually stepping on the scale.

What are the basics to muscle gain?

- Use of moderate or heavy weight through proper lifting form.

- Caloric surplus

What are the basics to power and strength?

- Use of very heavy weight through proper lifting form.

What are the basics to toning and weight loss?

- Caloric deficit

- Use of light weight combined with high intensity through proper lifting form.

I want to be an actor in Hollywood. Will having nice abbs help?

The look along with some talent significantly improves the chances of landing the audition.

Is it enough to just do lots of crunches and other abb exercises?

Concentration on abdominal exercises is tremendously beneficial. However, taking off the fat that covers the abdominal area is a multi-step process. You can have the most breathtaking abbs underneath the fat hidden away from the world and never get to show them. Focus on the whole program, not just abdominal exercises.

I have a full time job and other commitments. I'm not sure if I can do this.

Attitude is the driving factor that puts us in a state of victory or failure. If you doubt and think negative, you forfeit before making a single move. Stay positive and believe in yourself. Always.

I have almost no extra money for good healthy food, what should I do?

That's not an excuse. You can get ripped by shopping at the 99 cent store. Some of the key things you need that most 99 cent stores carry are:

- Clean frozen low sodium meats

- Vegetables

- Salad greens

- Plain oatmeal

- Brown rice

- Whole grain breads

- Low sodium seasoning

- Canned tuna

- Other clean foods on weekly sale

Any other suggestions?

You must be true to yourself and make the decision to stay committed before you start. As a personal trainer, I can comfortably state that one of the major problems as to why people do not achieve their goals is because they mentally do not have a solid foundation. Don't just jump in on impulse. Commit, then stick with it.

(Note) Earning those Hollywood abbs requires a long distance marathon runners mentality. It takes time. A sprinters mentality almost always fails. Gratification comes, but it's not instant.

CHAPTER 2
THE HOLLYWOOD ABBS COMMANDMENTS

And when the Greek abdominal gods gathered round, they decided to give the Hollywood abb commandments onto the Spartans. Not so much the Athenians.

1. **The way you think is the way you feel. Think positive, think abbs.**
2. **Follow the mirror, not the scale.**
3. **Eating clean food does not mean eating less.**
4. **Cardio, cardio and more cardio.**
5. **A cheat meal is not a cheat day.**
6. **If the body hurts, rest and recover. But always maintain a clean diet.**
7. **Use light to moderate free weights combined with high intensity.**
8. **Organization**
9. **Patience**
10. **Commitment**

1. **The way you think is the way you feel. Think positive, think abbs.**

For a moment reflect on your week. Were you positive all the time? Think back a bit further now into the past year. Could you have been more positive in some situations? In those past negative moments, if you reacted in a more positive way would that have helped you?

Every reaction /action we have to any situations influences the internal mood. The unfortunate part is, sometimes a single unpleasant moment may put a person in a negative state of mind for the entire day. That day then evolves into a concoction of disastrous behavior. If you want good looking abbs you must stay positive. Why?

Because eating a clean diet and training hard to get those abbs is not an easy task to achieve. The last thing that a person should do is break a healthy diet and consistent training when he or she is feeling bad due to some event that could have been tackled with the right attitude in the first place. If positive attitude is dominating your thoughts, you will not dwell on the small insignificant things that may hold you from those Hollywood abbs. Different events happen regularly in our daily life, these events set off chain reactions leading towards other events. As some say, when it rains it pours. If a distressing event dominates the tough process, the influenced person who is perusing the Hollywood abbs temporarily gives up or postpones the abdominal pursuit.

"Ahh what the hell, I'll just take the day off and come back to it tomorrow."

After some drinks and a greasy pizza, that person usually comes to a conclusion of "O crap what the hell did I do?" Then, as a reaction, that person kills him or herself by training extra hard, completely overtaxing the body. (Thinking that he or she can make up for the pizza and drinks). The impulsive reaction to stabilizing the damage leads to a quick burnout followed shortly by a climax of discomforting pain.

The thought of

"I need something sweet" follows. Then the action of eating something sweet as well. Followed by more "Pity" food.

(Note) Usually the body acts on what the mind focuses on.

(Note) When the body is in a state of pain, and low blood sugar, pity crap foods are in high demand.

This common scenario leads to a circular yoyo trap.

If the person had the right attitude in the first place, the low blood sugar, the binge and the circular pattern could have been avoided. Looking back, we can comfortably say that this scenario was triggered by some event to which the person reacted negatively. The negativity transitioned into a harmful action and so that person let go.

(Note) A positive attitude tramples over negative situations. If you don't stay positive, the Hollywood abbs will be but a dream. Positive attitude is like a shield that utilizes the inner voice inside your head and says

"You can do it, keep moving forward, thank you for overcoming that bump on the road."

2. Follow the mirror, not the scale.

Perhaps one of the most destructive and anti abb things someone can do is frequently check his or her weight. Are you trying to get your abbs out or are you trying to drop weight?
These are not same. To clear it up, low body fat is necessary to have the abbs out. But, weight loss does not necessarily mean that you will get your abbs out. Ever heard of the term "skinny fat person?"
Losing weight, if done improperly not only means getting rid of the fat. It also means losing muscle and slowing down the metabolism. To have those Hollywood abbs, muscle maintenance is required through healthy nutrition and resistance training. So?
So a person could drop only 10 lbs in 6 months while continuing to tone up and look better by the day. It's even possible to gain some weight back and still look fabulous.
A natural reaction people have to the scale is a straightforward one.
"Ah crap I just gained a pound this is horrible" or "YES! I just dropped two pounds this is great."
Do people randomly come up to you and ask how much you weight or do they say something like "Damn you look great." If in fact you do look great.
It's all about the final look. Not the final weight.
The mirror does not lie, but the scale is very deceiving. The scale only tells you a number. Not the body fat weight, not how much food and liquid is in your stomach and not how the weight is distributed on your body.
But, the mirror screams loudly some of the following at you.

1. **You have a long way to go!**
2. **You are making good progress**
3. **Ok you look good in these jeans**
4. **Good job you look terrific without clothes, keep it up.**
5. **It's time to walk on stage with those abbs bay! Good job!**

If you still insist on hopping on the scale, please do it no more than once a month. However, if you hop on the scale you are still technically breaking the second abb commandment. The Greek abdominal gods do frown upon that.

Long live Abdominus Greatus.

3. Eating clean food does not mean eating less.

A common step that people take when they want to get their Hollywood abbs out is significantly lower the caloric intake. If this action is maintained and the person works out, an adverse reaction may occur. By physically straining and starving the body, the metabolism says "You are crazy my friend, so I'm gonna slow down as long as you keep eating less. Both of us can play this less is best game."
The metabolism slows down as a response to insufficient fuel (food) and excessive body use (working out). It's a self-preservation safety mechanism.
None the less, through caloric deficit weight loss will occur. The problem is that this weight loss will be muscle and fat. As mentioned previously, the more muscle lost, the slower the metabolism functions. This is not a good thing.
So how does one combat this?
The person should eat frequent and healthy.
Eating frequent healthy meals allows that body furnace to keep burning hot and hold on to the muscle while shredding the fat.
For some reason people think if they stop eating food they will look great.
Not true.
Skinny flabby is not attractive. Lean and ripped is. Hollywood abbs are not flabby my friends.

The following is for example purposes only:

Bad Idea
Morning coffee (no significant food) [Did not fuel up].
Small lunch sandwich [Not enough fuel or protein to repair body tissues].
     Workout time
Medium size dinner (brown rice and a small piece of fish) [the body is starving at this point].

Good Idea
Meal 1) Oatmeal with fruit [just fuelled up for the day].
Meal 2) Small meat/chicken/fish meal with some greens and rice or small plain baked potato. [A little more fuel and protein].
Meal 3) Protein shake or small meat/chicken/fish meal with some greens [protein].
     Workout time
Meal 4) Protein shake or small meat/chicken/fish meal with some greens [protein].
Meal 5) Tuna salad. [protein].

"Eat frequent, small, quality meals. But, when all else fails, Mr. Protein shake to the rescue."

4. Cardio, cardio and more cardio.

The fourth Hollywood abbs Commandment is doing lots of cardio. Preferably a run with some hills after the training session. If the person has bad joints or other health problems that prevent him or her from running, an intense training circuit with lots of movement that does not hurt should provide a secondary alternative.

The fat blasting running approach works exceptionally well and for many it's a love hate relationship. At first comes the hate. Then when the abbs slightly start showing the love follows. Eventually, when the abbs are out entirely some say "Holy Zeus I love to run, I love my abbs, why did I not do this before?"

Why would anyone need the Stairmaster or the treadmill when running up and down hilly terrain with natural wind resistance is so much better. And no one said that you instantly start running ten miles a day. No one says that you hall ass fast when you start running. Hell, maybe a quarter mile walking is all someone can do in the beginning. The important thing is to build that stamina and remember the fourth abb commandment. Cardio is a daily thing, it's not a three times a week approach. Just be sure to stretch and have comfortable running shoes.

Some of you will break this commandment and use a cardio machine like the; Elliptical, Treadmill or the Stairmaster. All these things will work. But, try to get those runs in eventually. If you don't do cardio at all, with time you can still get those awesome Hollywood abbs out through diet and resistance training. I can tell you form experience that I rather have my abbs out 3 to 6 months sooner. That is why everyone healthy enough should cardio it up regularly.

The Hollywood abbs rating system for fat blasting cardio

1. Interval running with fast, moderate and slow speed. (Difficulty / very hard)

2. Interval running with fast and slow speed. (Difficulty / hard)

3. Stairmaster (Difficulty / hard)

4. Moderate speed running (Difficulty / moderate)

5. Slow long running (Difficulty / moderate)

6. Elliptical and treadmill machines (Difficulty / easy to moderate)

7. Stationary bike (Difficulty / easy)

8. Walking (Difficulty / easy)

Regardless what cardio level you start at, be sure to start.
This rating system many not be an accurate approach for all, but it still kicks ass.

5. A cheat meal is not a cheat day.
You know who you are when I say you are guilty of this.

"Oh like whatever, I'll just have this small brownie. " Three brownies later the binge monster manifests and takes possession. Then, lots of other junk goes down the hatch.

So how can the fifth Hollywood abb commandment aid?

Follow the following three steps in order.

Step one) Select a Friday, Saturday or Sunday night as the one cheat meal for the week.

Step two) Throw in 20-40 additional minutes of cardio that day.

Step three) Repeat the following 5 times if you ever want to chomp down on some unhealthy crap and it's not time for the cheat meal.

"I want to have my abbs out, I want to look and feel great. This decision I'm about to make eating crap food will set me back, and I know this. I will keep moving forward because I made a commitment. "

Welcome to the world of stunning abbs. If you do not pay the price you do not get the prize.

6. If the body hurts, rest and recover. But always maintain a clean diet.

There are times when a person can train for two weeks every day, not take a break and feel normal. However, there are also times when a person may workout for one day and then need two days off.

What does this all mean in the context of the big Hollywood abbs picture?

You must listen to your body. A pain there or a pain here is a good indication to take a break if you understand good pain and bad pain.

- Good pain- muscle soreness (most of the time you can work around or through this pain).
- Bad pain- strains, pulls, whining muscle pain from over use, joint pain etc. (A bad pain is an indication to take it easy)

If you sense that more than one day is necessary to recover, do not hesitate to take extra days off. A day off is a strategic retreat form the battlefield. Recover to come back strong again and win the war.

How do I strategically retreat?

1. Do not train for at least one day.
2. Do not eat crap foods on the day off.
3. Drink plenty of water.
4. If the body asks you for another day off, follow your gut and do so.
5. On the off day you might want to throw in a little more complex carbohydrates into the diet.

(Note) If you take a whole week off to recover and not eat crap food, you are still at 100%.

(Note) Lazy down time and recovery time are two different things. One is necessary, and the other one isn't. Take recovery time to recover, not lounge around a few extra days.

7. Use light to moderate free weights combined with high intensity.

In the process of slimming down and burning fat, it's not necessary to lift heavy. But, it is very helpful to lift with high intensively and light-weights. Believe it or not, after 50 consecutive repetitions, a light weight gets heavy fast.

What if I want to lift heavy?

Heavy lifting combined with high intensity training is not recommended because the person has less control over the heavy weight. If control is lost, safety goes out the window and injury is invited in. Always keep in mind that this is not a bodybuilding training approach. This is the Hollywood abdominal fat blasting approach.

---

8. Organization

Sometimes I think organization should be the first Hollywood abbs commandment. It's so crucial to stay organized that your overall success depends on it. Here are some steps you could take to make sure you are on top of things.

- Do the food shopping in advance.
- Make a list before bed time for the following day of things to do.
- Cross off the completed tasks from the list.
- Prepare or start to prepare meals in advanced. For example, you can broil 5 or 6 chicken breasts the night before, chop up some salad greens, make some brown rice and have canned tuna in water ready on the side just in case.
- Plan out the workouts in advance.
- Utilize the free time on non-training days towards something productive like not watching television for 3 hours straight.

(Note) Think of organization as a bridge. You can only train and burn fat on this bridge and nowhere else. If the bridge foundation is weak, the bridge will collapse.

9. Patience

I am truly sorry when I say that instant gratification and sexy Hollywood abbs are not the best of friends.

Why?

Because it takes iron clad patience to go through the Hollywood abbs journey. Getting those abbs out sort of works like this. Pretend that you are bicycling from Los Angeles to New York and there is no other means of transportation. You know for a fact that if you are patient you will get to your destination. You also know that getting to that destination takes time. By realizing the whole extent of the trip before you set off on the journey, you look at the whole picture form a realistic perspective. You enter into the right, long term mind set.

1. Instant sexy Hollywood abbs only exist through surgery or Photoshop.
2. If you are not taking the surgery rout, to speak like Yoda for a moment "Patience have, you must."

Thank you for your patience.

---

10. Commitment

Abbs are like a serious relationship. They require commitment. In this long term commitment, you face ups and downs. But, because of the serious nature of the relationship, the flaws are constantly worked on.

The Hollywood abbs commitment will test a person daily. If that person did not seriously think about the abb commitment it will be short lived. As in most new relationships, an experienced high is in the air (the honeymoon stage) form the training and a feeling of fulfillment. Then something happens and the commitment is broken. (This is where you cheated with crap food on your abbs). The pursuit of Hollywood abbs then stops with a period of mild depression.

"Why did I cheat? Why?"

A one night stand approach is for the weekend warrior. That is why weekend warriors almost never get those good looking abbs out from underneath the fat. But, if you do not cheat and make the relationship work, the abbs will show you love.

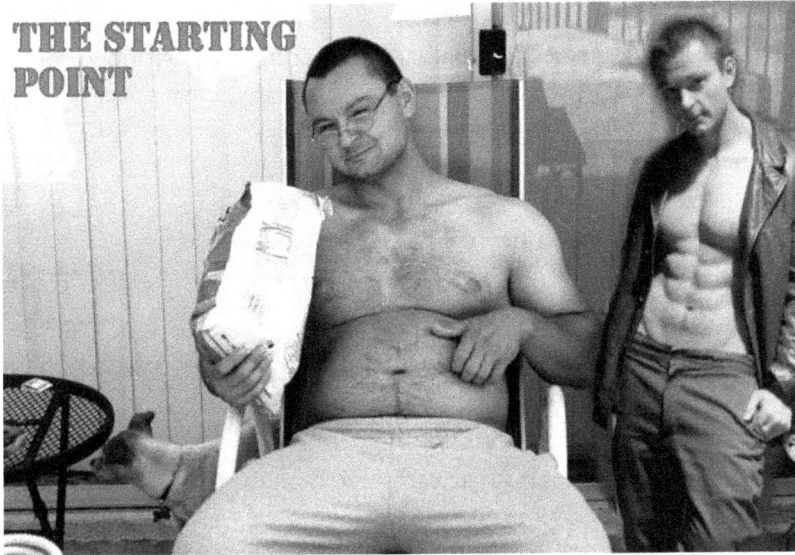

THE STARTING POINT

CHAPTER 3
THE STARTING POINT

Every individual who decides to go on the Hollywood abbs journey must first realistically asses his or her overall situation. The person should look at things like:

- Current health
- Commitments (job, family, work, school, etc…)
- Goals
- Who are the birds of feather you flock together with?
  (Positive vs negative influences)

Once some basic categories are looked over, you can (with more accuracy) find your overall starting point. Not to understand the starting foundation upon which you will sculpt your abbs is like jumping without looking on top of a cliff. For the following, I will use myself as an example. This should help you realistically asses your own starting point.

Originally when I wrote my first fitness book I was in top shape with fat free abbs. Then, for stupid reasons of neglect it all changed. I completely stopped training and started drinking lots of beer as well as eating greasy, sugary, fatty processed foods. This was done in large, unhealthy portions. For about seven months, I followed a horrible daily ritual.

- Oven pizza at least once a day.
- Online video gaming for 6 to 8 hours per day conquering evil in Diablo 3.
- Drinking lots of beer with salty chips.
- Netflix galore along with a sugar loaded drink and buttered up popcorn to wrap up the night by 3am.
- Sleeping in past one pm.
- Starting the day with a high sugar caffeinated energy drink to wake up.

(Note) One regular 16 oz sugar energy drink contains 70 grams of sugar. That's 17.5 teaspoons of sugar.

For a long time, I did not leave the house unless it was to get more pizza or beer. At 250lbs of crap, I felt the fat jiggle stomach dance on every step. To make it worse, walking to a local 7-11 across the street I hurt my knee and that made me move even less for a few weeks. After each meal, I had to take a nap, and there was no contemplation about it. It was nap time or the end of the world.

I do not know how many other average people can say that their starting point was worse than mine. I am sure that some individuals have it much worse, that is not an argument I am making. But, In general health speaking terms I was f***d.

My life commitments at the starting point were few. I got lucky on that one. Other than a part time marketing job form home and basic bills I had no other obligations. If you have numerous obligations be sure to follow Hollywood abbs commandment number 8. Without it, you will be in a world of troubled stress.

I have a few good friends and many chill drinking friends too. At the starting point, I slowly backed off from the bad influences. Let me tell you, some chill friends will ruin and bring you down, and they won't do it on purpose. They will do it because it's in their nature to party. You need to see that ahead of time to know how to avoid putting yourself in a situation full of unhealthy temptation.

Another important thing to consider is that we all need to speak our mind and share certain things with people. Know who those positive people are. Know who will support you and listen to you when the pain kicks in. At the starting point, it's not a cake walk. A good supportive friend is of much help. A good friend influences you to keep moving forward.

For me, the tipping point came when the power went out, and Netflix with Diablo 3 ceased to function. I took a long walk and decided that I was going to write another book on fitness. The rest was sweat, pain and history.

1. Think about the difficulties you will encounter outside of training and how you can prepare for those difficulties prior to the Hollywood abbs journey. Do not just jump in without thinking about the things that may derail you.
2. If you have the opportunity to do a health checkup including blood work, do it. The last thing you want to do is start training and not know if any health issues should be taken care of first.
3. If you have some physical limitations it does not mean you can't maintain a positive attitude.
   (Note) One of my friends is paralyzed from the waist down, and he is ripped to shreds.
4. Hollywood abbs require the person to go above and beyond the standard approach of training. Yes, you will probably start slow and build up to more difficult routines. Just be sure to review and follow the Hollywood abbs commandment number 10.

Regardless from where you start
Regardless how long it takes
Regardless if you have or do not have support from friends and family,
start.
If you succumb to the belief that it is not possible, then you fail before you
begin.

Tomorrow is always tomorrow.
Live today.
Train today.
Push yourself today.
Commit today.
You don't have to be just average today.
Eventually, one day today, you will thank yourself.
Yes you can.

Thank you

CHAPTER 4
A LOOK AT A POSITIVE WEEK

One day before starting

Sunday July 8th 2012
Tomorrow the training starts but today I'm a fat ass. This is why:

11:45 am-breakfast at the local diner (bacon cheeseburger combo) with an energy drink and a 32 oz soda. (No joke)
12:30 pm-lunch   (medium pepperoni pizza) with an energy drink..
10:00 pm-dinner (9 beers, bag of chips, garlic bread sticks).
11:00 pm-dinner#2 (Mexican fast food tacos, rice, beans, burrito combo).

Today's activities (the standard Sunday)

Watching online movies at home
Drinking with friends
Diablo 3 online gaming (7 hours plus)

On day one, I decided that the 10th Hollywood abbs commandment was to be flipped on like a light switch and stay in the on position. Permanently.

Monday July 9th 2012 Day 1
Today's food

7:30 am - oatmeal (plain) 1 cup/ with blueberries on top
10:30 am - protein shake
1:00 pm - grilled chicken breast, small baked potato, asparagus, (fish oil and a multi vitamin)
4:00 pm- grilled chicken breast, small baked potato, asparagus, (fish oil, multi vitamin and glucosamine)
(5pm-7:40 pm training time)
7:45 pm - post workout protein shake
10:00 pm - canned tuna and a spinach salad

Today's activities
Work
Looked for a second part time job.
Training

Notes from day 1
Holy crap! I just got done training and I already want to quit. I kid you not; the first thought out of my head after I finished working out was to eat something unhealthy. The two plus hours of training wiped me out. But, the beauty of experience is that I know for a fact that soon this F*** pain will continuously decrease. Either I will beat the pain, or it will beat me.

Word of advice #1
Some people have an (ON and OFF) switch when it comes to eating clean and working out. Most of us can't turn that switch on instantly. To prevent a burn out start slow if you must, but remain consistent. Remember to follow the Hollywood abbs Commandments.

Motivation from Ilya
The starting point (Day 1) is no fun. This is where everything may start to hurt. Sometimes certain body parts scream at you. However, the good news is that it eventually gets easier. You might be a long way from those Hollywood abbs. But, if you stay the course, victory shall be yours.

Tuesday July 10th 2012 <u>Day 2</u>
Today's food

7:30 am - oatmeal (plain) 1 cup/ with strawberries on top
10:30 am - protein shake
1:00 pm - grilled chicken breast, brown rice (cup), broccoli, (fish oil, multi vitamin and glucosamine)
4:00 pm- grilled chicken breast, brown rice (cup), broccoli, (fish oil and a multi vitamin)
(5:15 pm-7:00 pm <u>training time</u>)
7:05 pm - post workout protein shake
10:00 pm - canned tuna and a spinach salad

Today's activities
Work
Second job interview
Training

Notes from day 2
You have no idea how bad I didn't want to train today. But, I did. Now I feel great. It was more of a psychological thing than a physical pain. Even though the muscle soreness is kicking in from yesterday.

<u>Word of advice #2</u>
If it was easy, everyone would have sculpted abbs. But, if you are committed to training, the journey is much easier. Stay committed to your goals. Do not derail from the path of Hollywood abbs.
(Hollywood abbs commandment # 10)

<u>Motivation from Ilya</u>
The average person is capable of doing a lot more than what he or she thinks. Don't let negative people bring you down. Don't let unwholesome thoughts drag you down. Don't let excuses come between you and your goals. You are capable of a lot more. Five years from now do you want to look back and say <u>I should have,</u> or <u>I did</u>?
In life, to be in the audience as a spectator is easy.
To be on stage is not.

Wednesday July 11th 2012 <u>Day 3</u>
Today's food

7:30 am - oatmeal (plain) 1 cup/ with raspberries on top
10:30 am - protein shake
1:00 pm - grilled chicken breast, 2 small yams, broccoli, (fish oil, multi vitamin and glucosamine)
4:00 pm- grilled chicken breast, 2 small yams, broccoli, (fish oil and a multi vitamin)
(5pm -7:40 pm <u>training time</u>)
7:45 pm - post workout protein shake
10:00 pm - canned tuna and a spinach salad

Today's activities
Work.
Went out to look for a second part time job
Training

Notes from day 3
Day one was not easy, day two was just as bad. Today I'm in sore discomforting physical pain, but mentally I feel accomplished. Because of clean eating for the last three days, I can see in the mirror that some excessive water and bloat dropped from the body. It's a bit easier to move around. Trying to be careful and not hurt the knee again. I was going to apply the Hollywood abbs commandment # 6 today and take a day off. But, I still trained and mainly concentrated on (slow jogging and abbs).

<u>Word of advice #3</u>
Stay hydrated and keep a bottle of water handy. In the car, at home and at work. Dehydration is not something you want to experience, especially when in training for Hollywood Abbs.

<u>Motivation from Ilya</u>
Quit... Because not everyone wants Hollywood abbs
Quit... Because not everyone wants to look good
Quit... Being like everyone

Thursday July 12th 2012 <u>Day 4</u>
Today's food

7:30 am - oatmeal (plain) 1 cup/ with blueberries on top
10:30 am - protein shake
1:00 pm - grilled tilapia, half avocado, brown rice, broccoli, (multi vitamin and glucosamine)
4:00 pm- grilled tilapia, half avocado, brown rice, broccoli, (multi vitamin)
(5 pm -7:40 pm <u>training time</u>)
7:45 pm - post workout protein shake
10:00 pm - canned tuna and a spinach salad

Today's activities
Work
Training
Started reading a new book/play: Long Day's Journey Into Night

Notes from day 4
Feeling slightly tiered due to additional hours put in at work. The back is in serious pain (muscle soreness).

<u>Word of advice #4</u>
The stress of work and life itself has a tendency to pop into our heads and cause inconvenient thoughts. Just because something thought provoking is going on at work or home, does not give you a free pass to skip a work out session or eat something unhealthy (Hollywood abbs commandment #1). Just a little bad food every day keeps the Hollywood abbs away. Remember that.

<u>Motivation from Ilya</u>
You have the option to reward yourself with a drink or a small unhealthy meal on a Friday or a Saturday. Having a cheat meal once or twice a week is undoubtedly, positively ok. The question is, are you strong enough not to. You think king Leonidas cheated? The power of 300 is in you. If you want Hollywood abbs bad enough that is (Hollywood abbs commandment #5).

(Note) If you do go out and cheat, try to select a healthier option from the menu.
(Warning) When you eat clean, alcohol hits harder and faster. Be careful.

Friday July 13th 2012 Day 5
Today's food

7:30 am - oatmeal (plain) 1 cup/ with strawberries on top
10:30 am - protein shake
1:00 pm – lean ground turkey, half avocado, brown rice, broccoli, (fish oil, multi vitamin and glucosamine)
4:00 pm- lean ground turkey, half avocado, brown rice, broccoli, (fish oil and a multi vitamin)
(5 pm-7:40 pm training time)
7:45 pm - post workout protein shake
10:00 pm - canned tuna and a spinach salad

Today's activities
Work.
Got a second part time morning job.
Training

Notes from day 5
The legs hurt and the arms are annihilated.
This whole eating clean and training routine is developing into a habit.
Some friends went out for some drinks and invited me. Before I always said yes, today it was a no. Maybe in a few weeks.

Word of advice #5
Develop a habit of saying NO to things that harm your goals. Sometimes sacrifices are necessary.

Motivation from Ilya
Alcohol is one of those things many of us like. Unfortunately abbs and alcohol do not mix. If you want those Hollywood abbs, alcohol will have to wait.

Saturday July 14th 2012 <u>Day 6</u>
Today's food

7:30 am - oatmeal (plain) 1 cup/ with blueberries on top
8:20 am - 10:00 am <u>training time</u>
10:30 am - protein shake
1:00 pm – lean ground turkey, half avocado, brown rice, broccoli, (fish oil, multi vitamin and glucosamine)
4:00 pm- grilled salmon, half avocado, brown rice, broccoli, (fish oil and a multi vitamin)
7:00 pm – grilled chicken with asparagus
10:00 pm- large bowl of fresh strawberries

Today's activities
Training
Yard work
Washed the car
Grilled up food in the back yard
Movie: Knight at the Roxbury "And I was all like, Emilio!"

Notes from day 6
Tiered from the week of working out but not exhausted. One of my friends decided to train with me today and as a result got a dreadful headache. I told him he needs to gradually build up and apply the Hollywood abbs commandments instead of showing off for the ladies. He will probably not train with me anymore. His overall foundation and commitment is somewhat weak. (Hollywood abbs commandment #8).

<u>Word of advice #6</u>
Listen to your body very carefully. For example if your shoulders hurt, don't train them that day. Focus more on other body parts. If you feel like you are out of energy, eat more. If you feel lousy, slow down and go easy on the weights. Remember, sometimes feeling lousy, is a masked excuse for feeling lazy.

<u>Motivation from Ilya</u>
Saturday is when all the weekend warriors pile into the gym. Want to get ahead? Train no less than five times per week. Think you can't do it? Ok, then someone else will.
Never give up on your goals.
Never give up on your dreams.

Sunday July 15th 2012 <u>Day 7</u>
Today's food

7:30 am - oatmeal (plain) 1 cup/ with blueberries on top

8:50 am - 9:30am training time (just a slow jog)

9:30 am - protein shake

11:00 pm – lean ground turkey, half avocado, brown rice, broccoli, (fish oil, multi vitamin and glucosamine)

2:00 pm- grilled salmon, half avocado, brown rice, broccoli, (fish oil and a multi vitamin)

5:00 pm - grilled chicken with asparagus

8:00 pm - canned tuna and a spinach salad

10:00 pm- large bowl of fresh blueberries

Today's activities
Training

Did some food shopping for the next week.

Grilled up food in the back yard.

Finished reading the book I started this week.

Movie - Amadeus

Weekly Review
Monday- My fat ass started moving

Tuesday - My fat ass is in pain

Wednesday- My fat ass is even in more pain

Thursday - I can see that some excess water has dropped from my body

Friday - Five days into it, feeling tiered but motivated

Saturday - The craving for junk food is diminishing

Sunday – A feeling of overall completion

Week one was a rough week. But I jumped into this whole thing with structure and the Hollywood abbs commandments behind my back. If you review week one carefully, you will see that everything was organized. Being organized (Hollywood abbs commandment # 8) helps in general no matter what you do. Also, this week I broke the pattern of not going out with friends and getting hammered or eating crap food. The most difficult part was the food. But now that I think about it, I actually saved money eating clean. Grilling up chicken and fish is very appetizing. The sizzle and the smell of grilled food is an experience I look forward to now. Along with getting the abbs out, I will become a back yard grill master in no time.

Can't wait for Monday.

CHAPTER 5
STRETCHING

When training or working out, no one is immune to the possibility of injury. The best thing we can do is lessen those chances of injury. How can we do that?
By stretching.
You are more than welcome to incorporate your own stretches in addition to the stretches presented in this chapter.

(Note) Always, always, always warm up for a few minutes before stretching.
A few minutes of running in place or a slow jog prior to stretching is a must.

Sequence of daily training events.
1. 5 minute warm up (get the blood and the oxygen moving)
2. Perform some basic stretches
3. Resistance training
4. Cardio

(Note) Do not neglect to stretch and warm up. From experience, I know that some will simply skip the stretching portion and go right into the workout. Not a good idea.

The following pages in this chapter are the suggested stretches to perform prior to training.

Brittni Johnson

Standing side bends

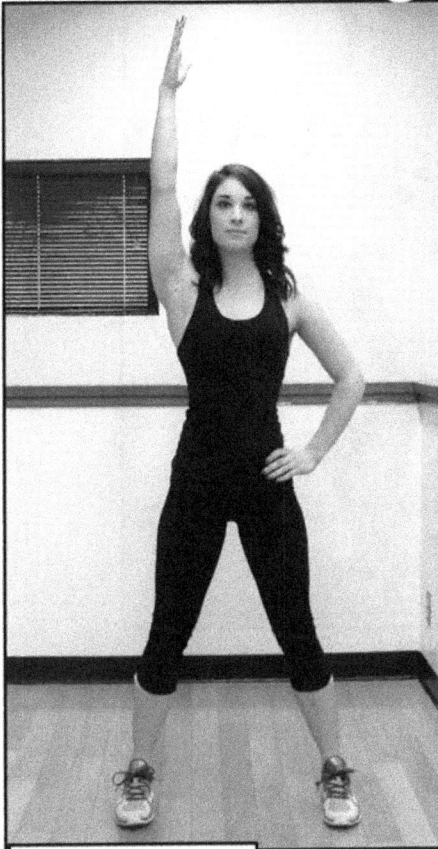

Starting position

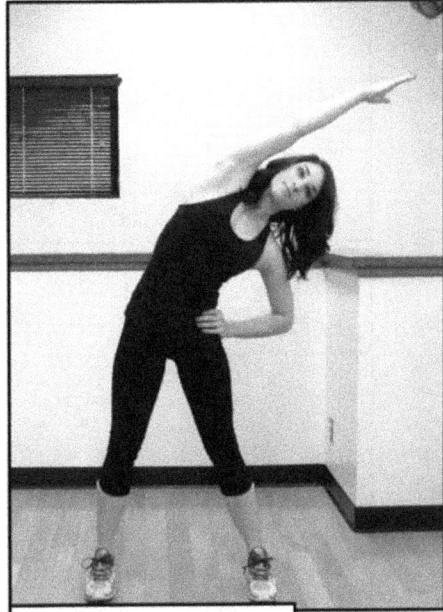

Ending position

1) Stand straight with the legs positioned apart.
2) Lift one hand straight up and place the other hand on the hip.
3) On the exhale, lean over to the side opposite of the extended hand and hold the stretch.

(Stretch target / trunk, obliques, inner thighs)

Back of the thigh and glute stretch

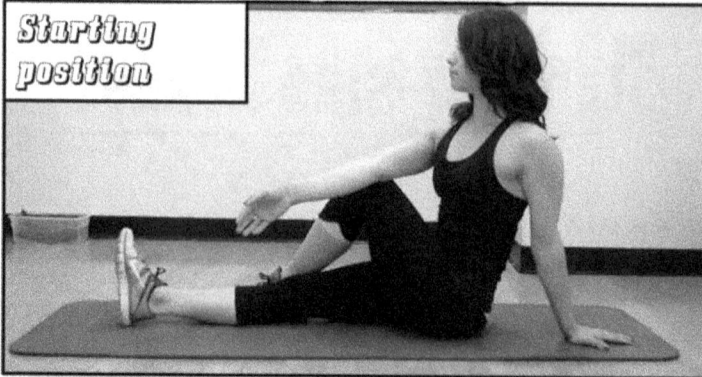

Starting position

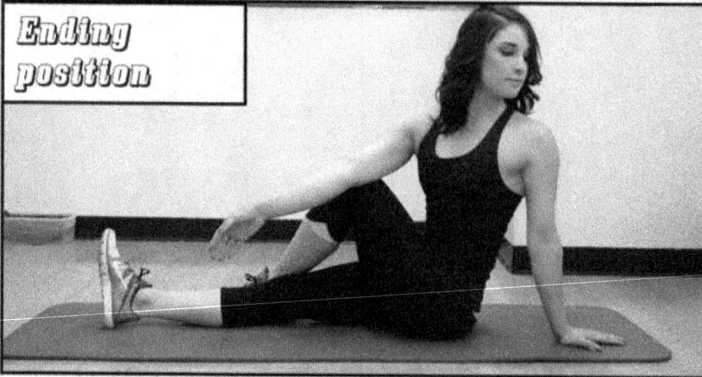

Ending position

1) Sit down on a flat surface with one leg extended forward and the other crossed over.
2) Place an opposite side elbow to the leg firmly behind the knee. Place the other hand on the ground for support.
3) On the exhale, twist away from the knee and apply pressure with the elbow.
   (Stretch target / glutes)

Seated hamstring stretch

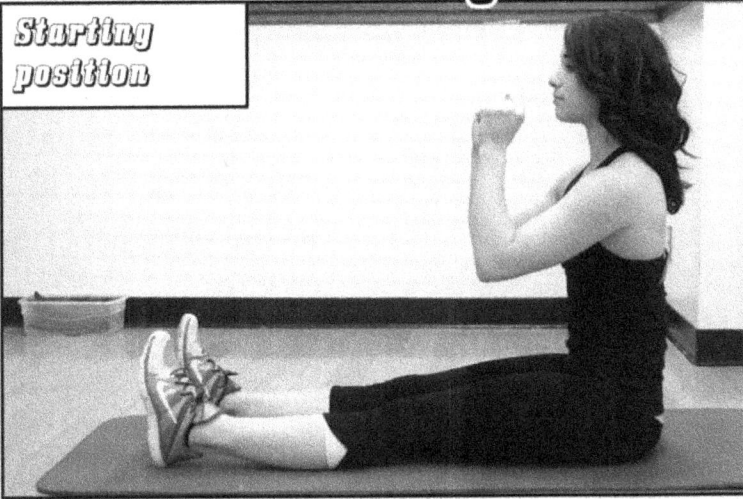

Starting position

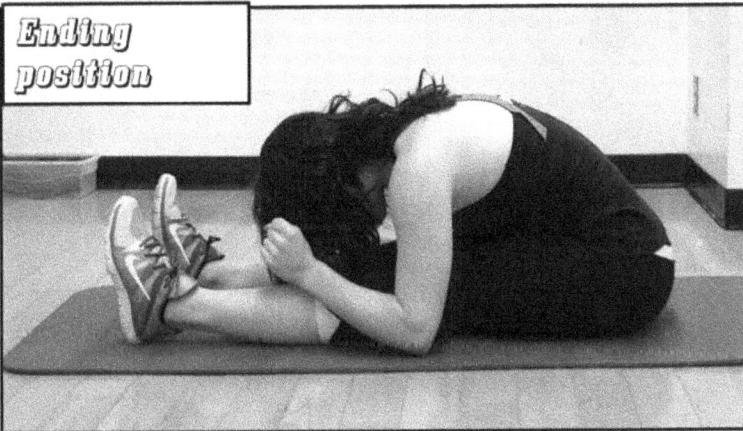

Ending position

1) Sit down on a flat surface with both legs extended forward and arms bent.
2) On the exhale, lean forward and try to make contact between the elbows and the knees. If you are flexible, try to make contact with the ground.
(Stretch target / hamstrings)

Standing quad stretch

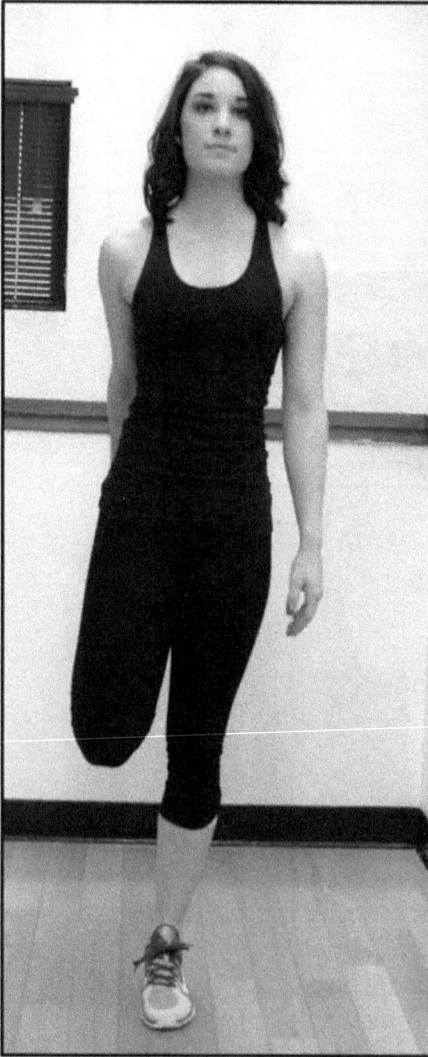

1) Stand straight balanced on one leg and hold the other leg at the ankle.
2) On the exhale, apply pressure to the ankle and pull the leg slightly back.
(Stretch target / quads)

Hip flexor and calf stretch

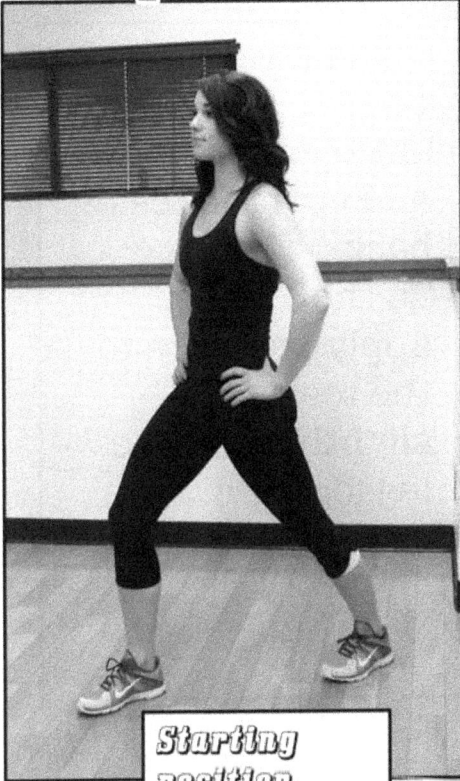

Starting position

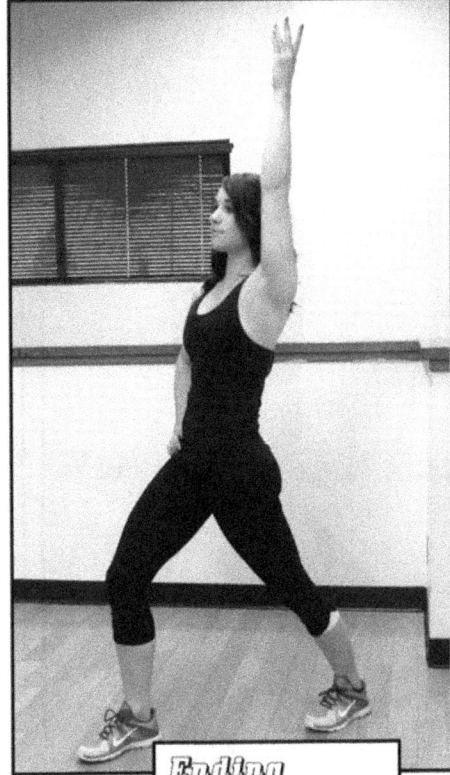

Ending position

1) Lunge forward with one leg. Keep the back leg straight.
2) Lift the opposite side arm to the front leg straight up.
3) On the exhale, lean back.
(Stretch target / hip flexors and calves)

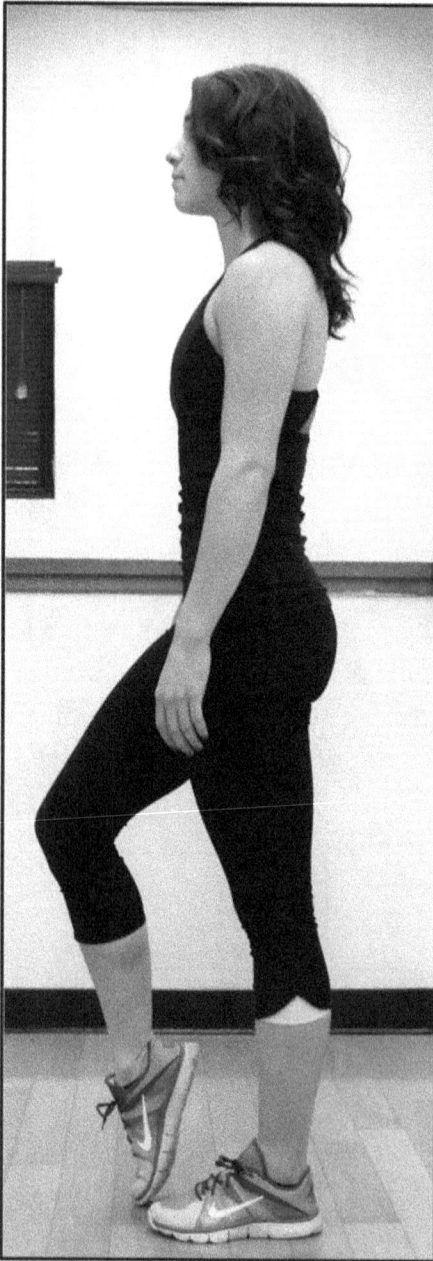

Standing shin stretch

1) Stand straight with one leg in the front.
2) Lift the front leg up and curl the toes back.
3) On the exhale, apply pressure to the toes and slightly push the leg forward.
(Stretch target / shins)

Starting position

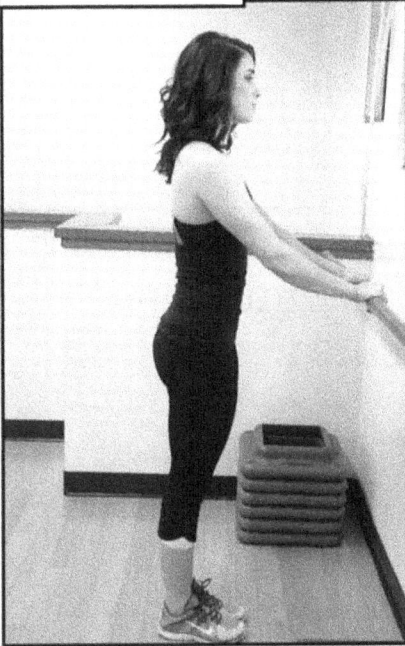

Back stretch

Ending position

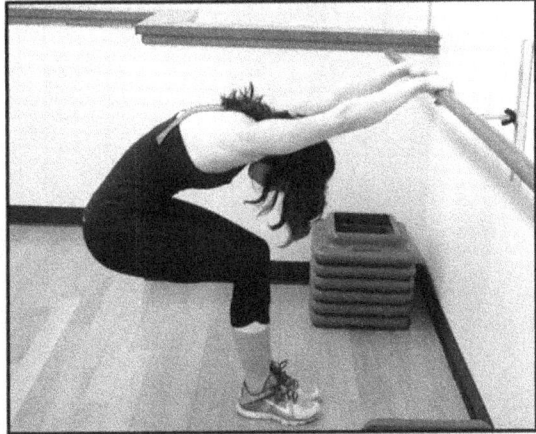

1) Grab hold of a wall, tree or a pole with both hands.
2) On the exhale, pull back and bend the knees.
(Stretch target / lats)

Back of the arm stretch

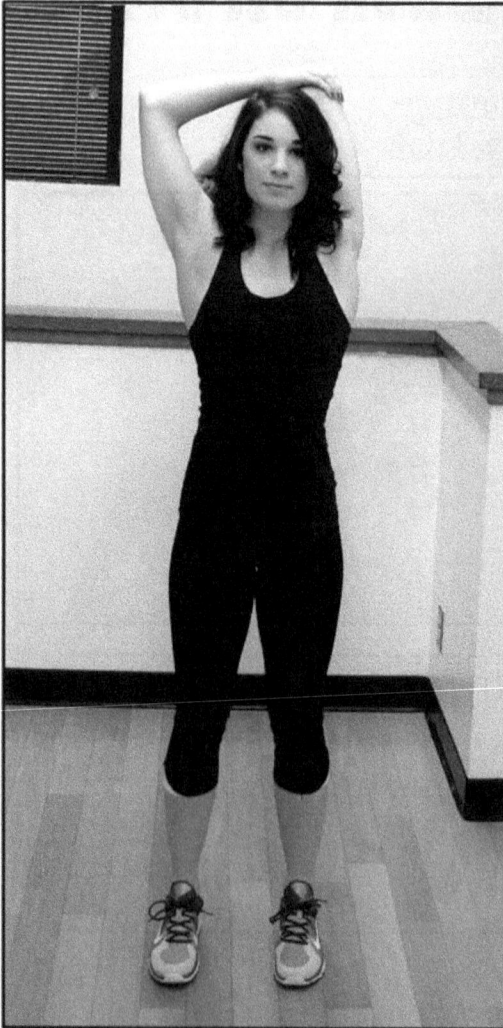

1) Place one arm behind the head and bend it.
2) On the exhale, with the opposite hand, apply pressure to the elbow.
(Stretch target / triceps)

Shoulder stretch

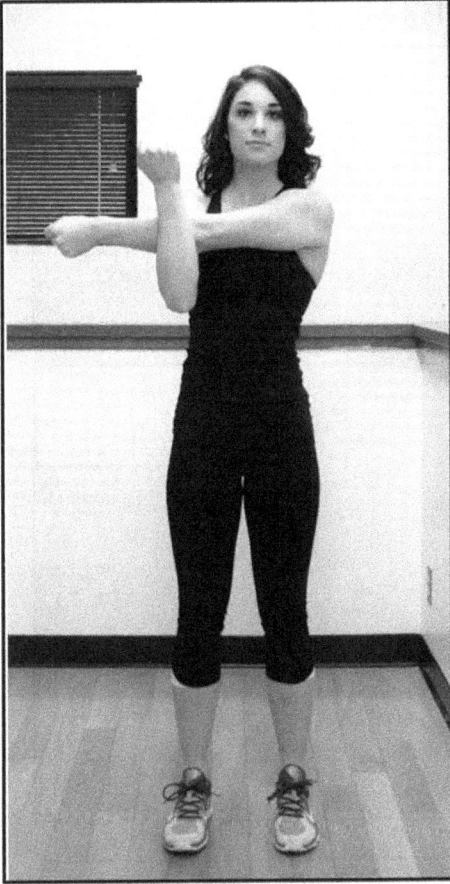

1) Position one arm across the chest.
2) On the exhale, apply pressure to the elbow with the other arm.

(Stretch target /deltoids)

Prone abb stretch

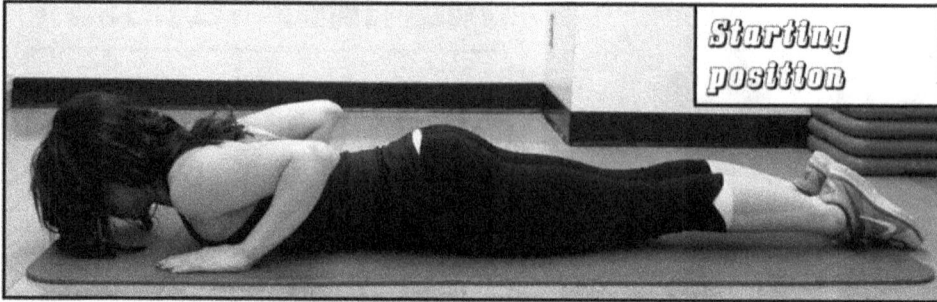

Starting position

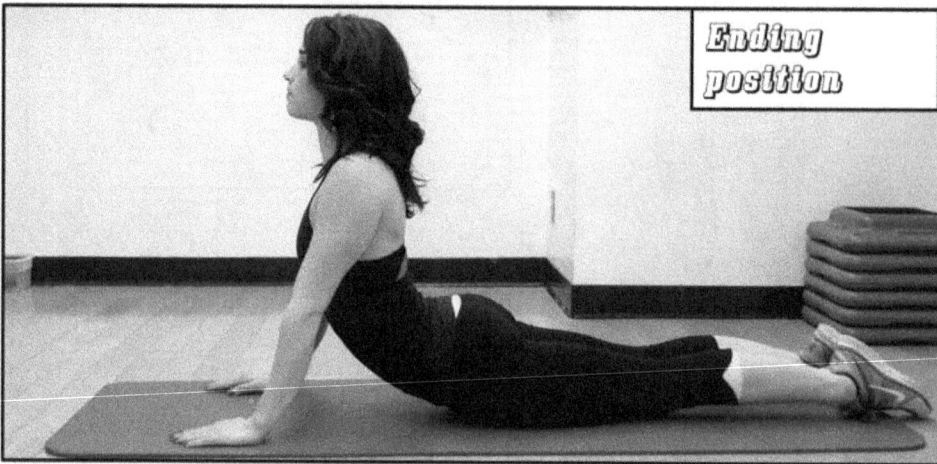

Ending position

1) Lay down flat on the floor and place both hands on the sides of the chest.
2) On the exhale, lift the upper body. (Stretch target / abbs)

Standing lat and abb stretch

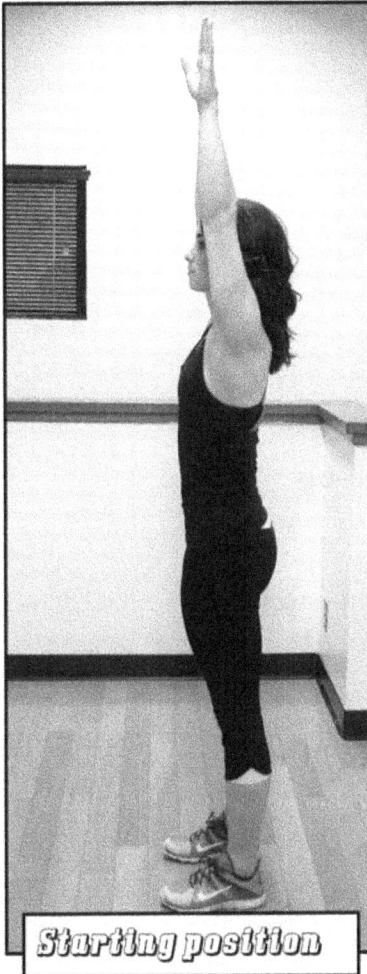

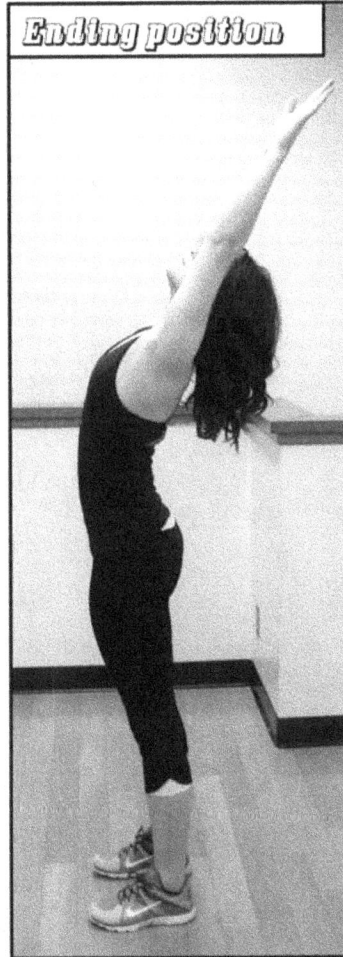

Ending position

Starting position

1) Position the legs at a wide stance and lift both arms up.
2) On the exhale, slightly lean back.
   (Stretch target / lats and abbs)

CHAPTER 6
THE BASICS WITHOUT WEIGHTS

The information from this chapter as well as the next will be combined into a program. Think of this chapter and the next as the basic training foundation for your Hollywood abbs journey.

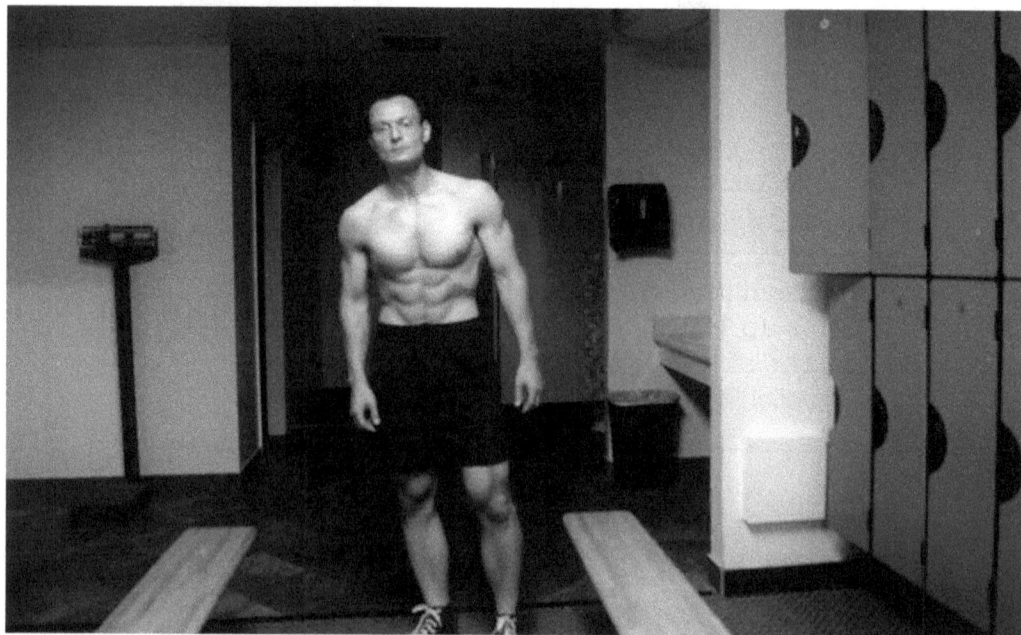

Shoulder holds

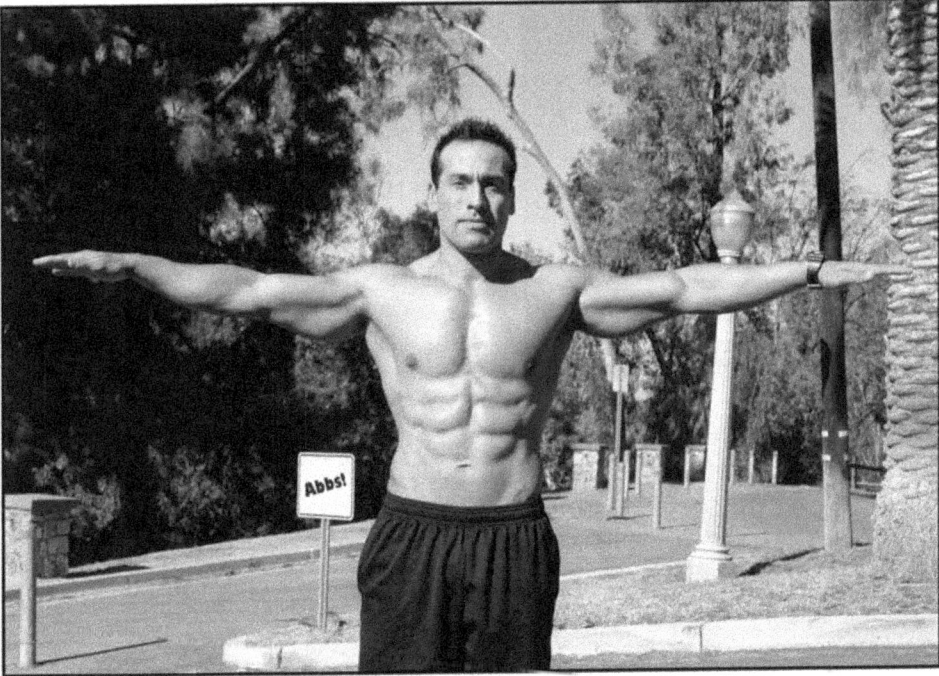

Stand straight with the arms
extended. Keep the palms faced
down. The abbs should be tight at all
times.
(Muscle target / deltoids)

Single side wall pulls

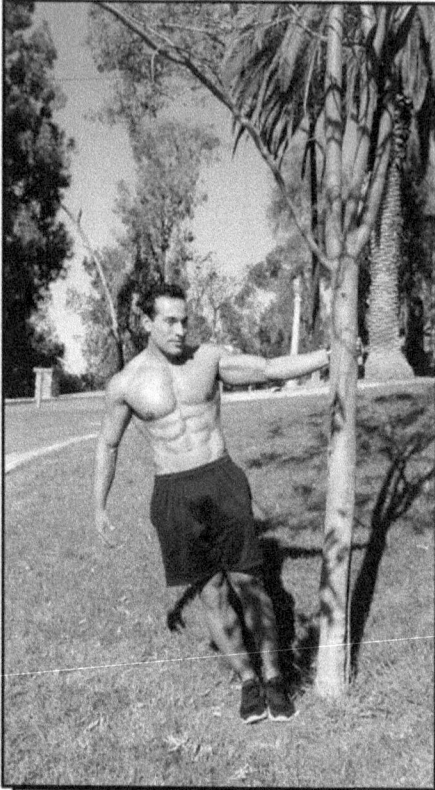

Starting position

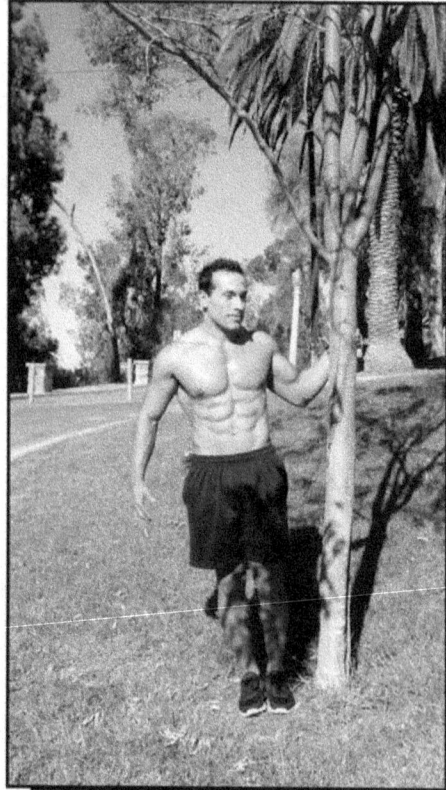

Ending position

1) Firmly take hold of a pole, tree or side of a wall and lean back on an angle.
2) On the exhale, contract the bicep and pull the body towards the hand that is holding on. Always keep the body straight and the abbs tight. (Muscle target / biceps and forearms)

Wide overhand bar pulls

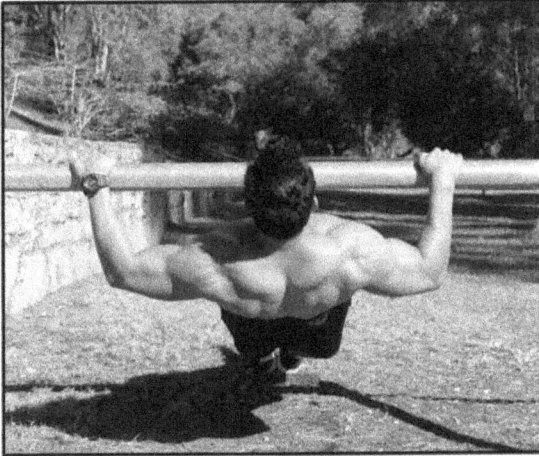

1) Grab on to a bar with a wide overhand grip.
2) On the exhale, contract the biceps, pull the chest towards the bar and bring the shoulder blades together.
3) On the inhale, lower the body back down to full arm extension.
(Muscle target / back and biceps)

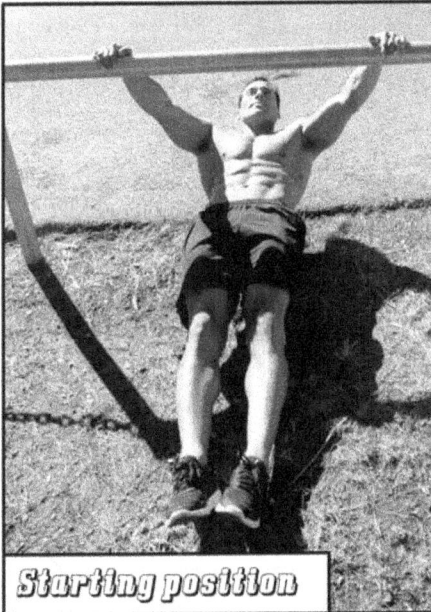

Starting position

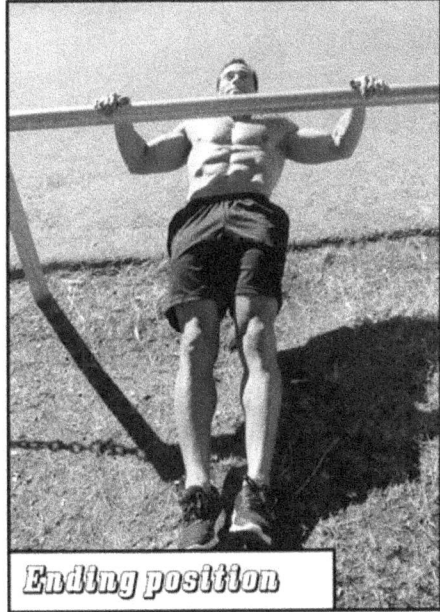

Ending position

Underhand bar pulls

Starting position

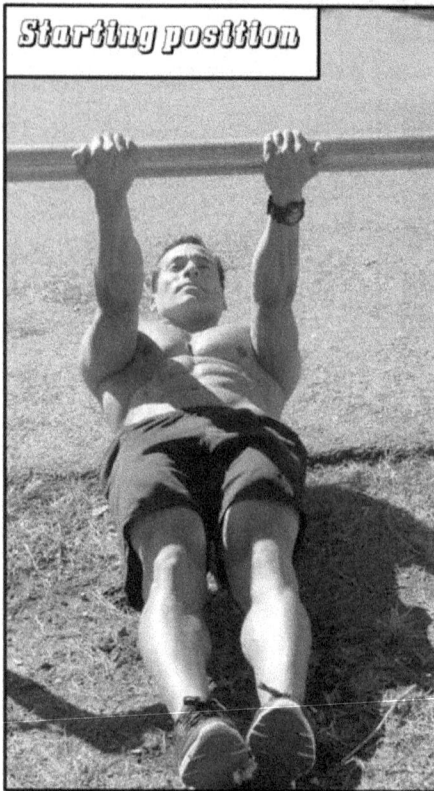

Ending position

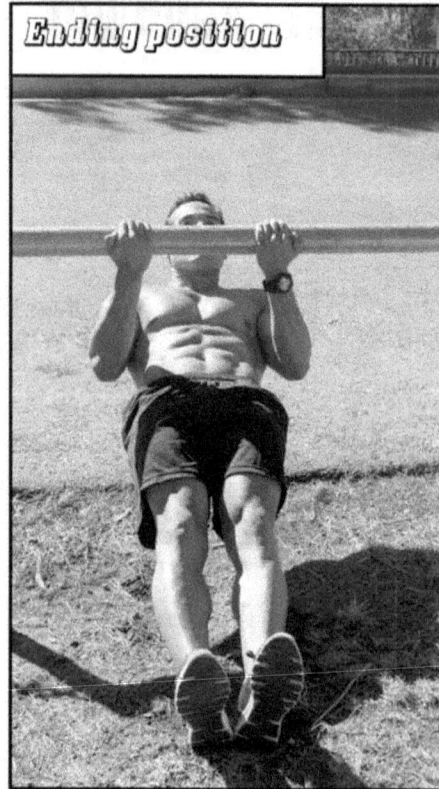

1) Grab on to a bar with an underhand grip. Keep the body straight and the abbs tight.

2) On the exhale, contract the biceps, pull the chest towards the bar and bring the shoulder blades together.

3) On the inhale, lower the body back down to full arm extension.

(Muscle target / back and biceps)

Staandard Pushups

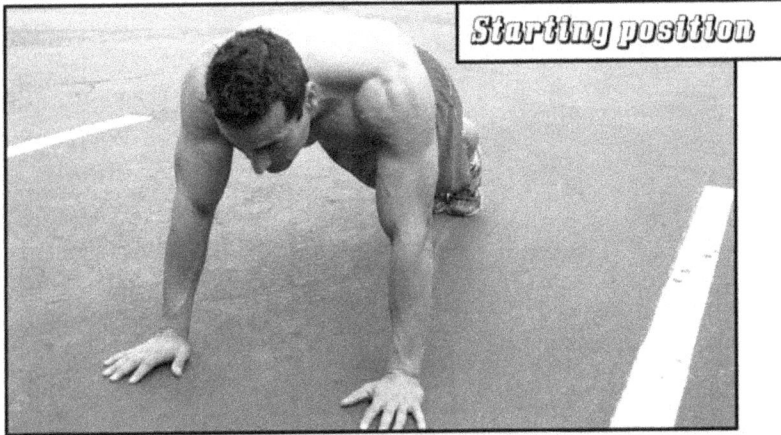

Starting position

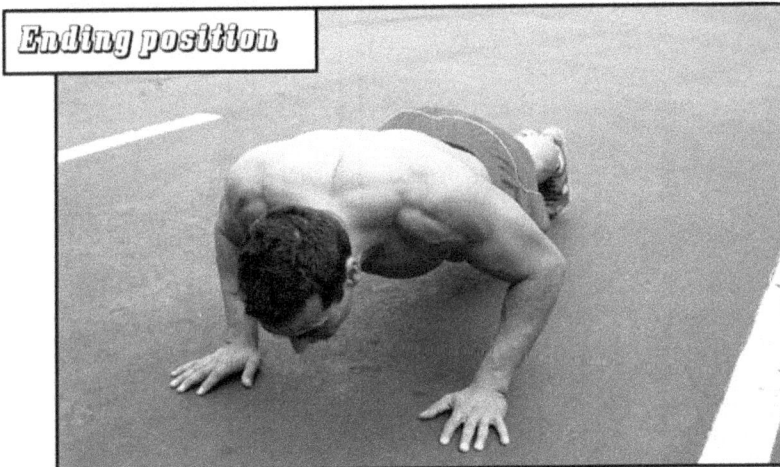

Ending position

1) On the inhale, come down towards the ground and feel a stretch in the chest.
2) On the exhale, push back up and flex the chest.

(Muscle target / Chest and triceps)

Wide pushups

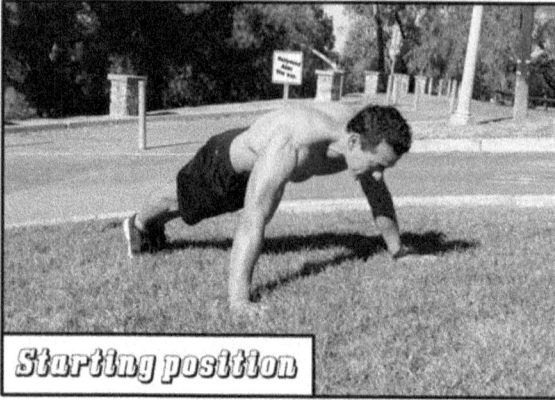

Starting position

1) From a standard pushup position, place the hands wide apart.
2) On the inhale, come down towards the ground and feel a stretch in the chest.
3) On the exhale, push back up.

(Muscle target / chest and triceps)

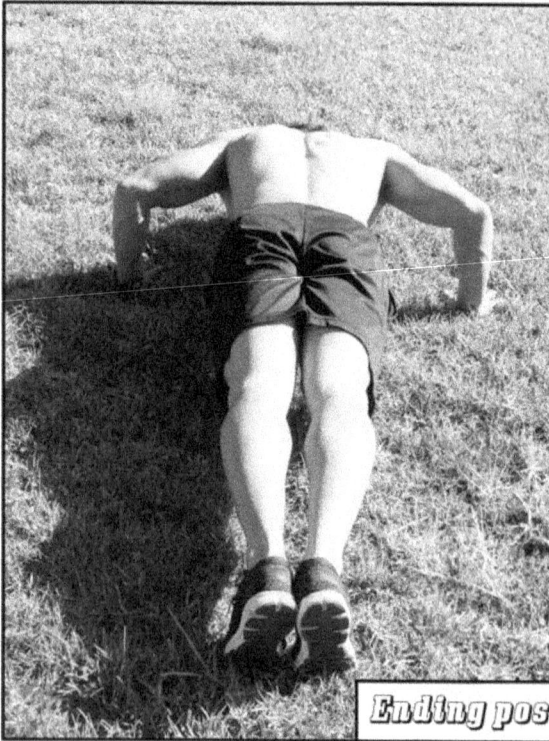

Ending position

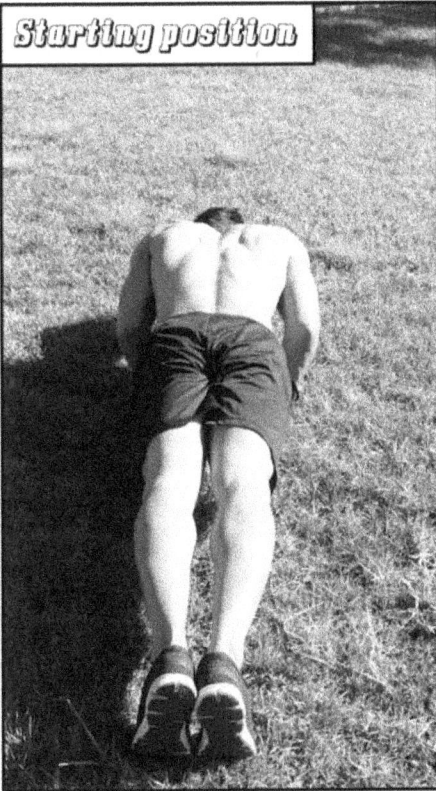

Starting position

Close pushups

A) Place the palms about a foot apart from each other.
B) Keep the abdominals tight.

1) As you are lowering the body towards the ground, inhale and slowly slide the elbows along the sides of the back.
2) On the exhale, slowly push back up. Do not lock out the arms at the top.
(Muscle target / triceps)

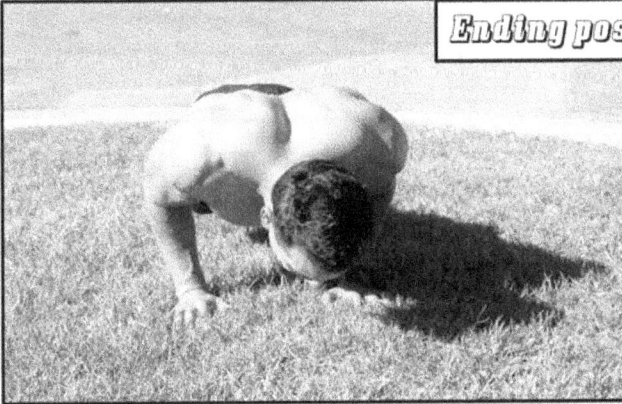

Ending position

Sumo squats

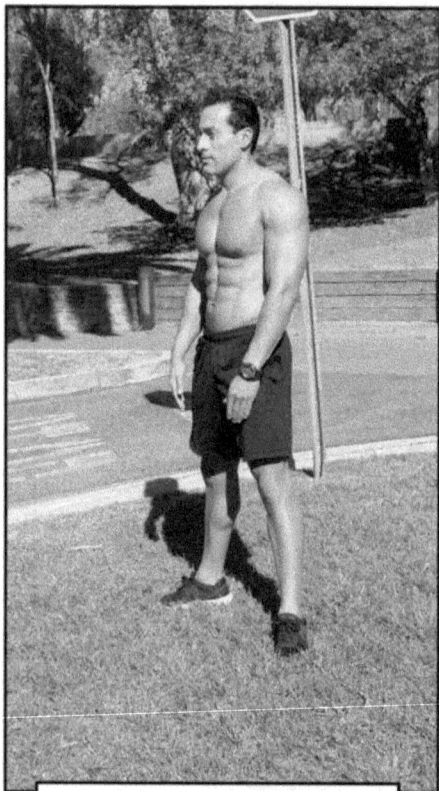

Starting position

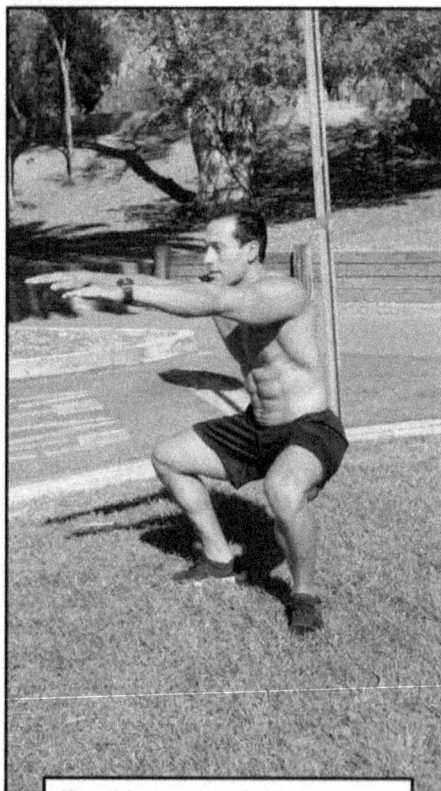

Ending position

1) Stand straight with the legs positioned wide apart. Keep the toes pointing outward.
2) On the inhale, squat down.
3) On the exhale, come back up.
(Muscle target / quads, hams and glutes)

Parallel close squats

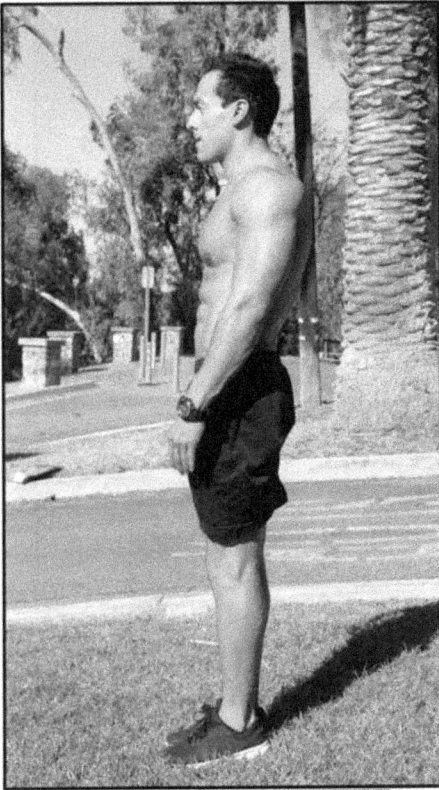

Starting position

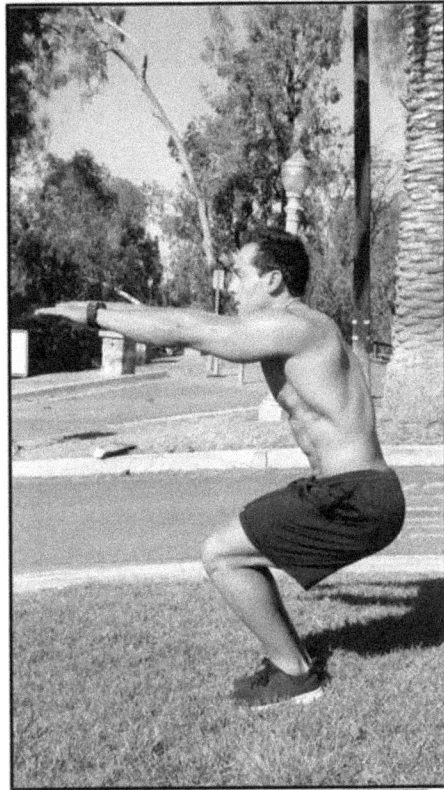

Ending position

1) Stand straight with the arms on the sides relaxed and the thighs touching.
2) On the inhale, squat down and lift the arms forward. Keep the abbs tight.
3) On the exhale, come back up to the starting position.
(Muscle target / quads)

Standing lower back extensions

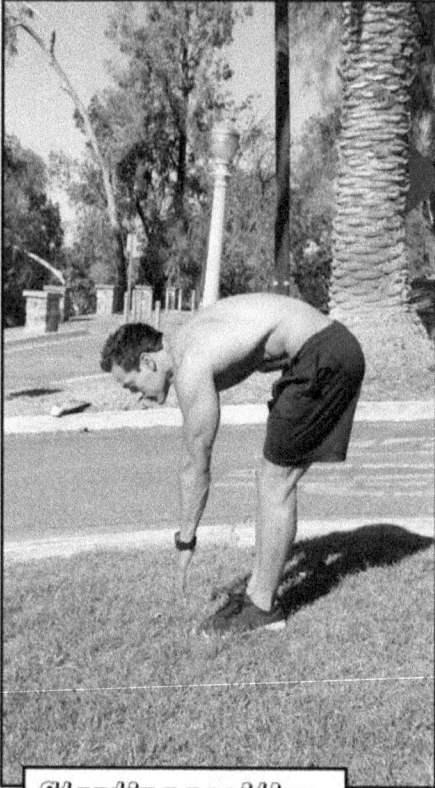

Starting position

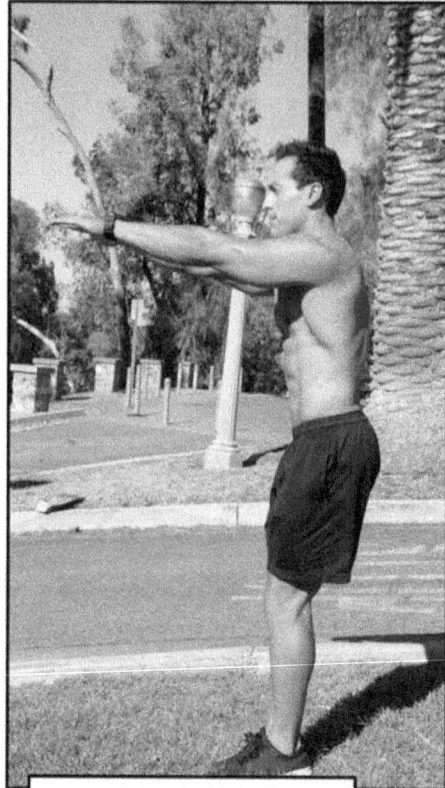

Ending position

1) Start out by reaching down towards the toes with the arms extended.
2) On the exhale, come up and flex the lower back. Do not change the position of the arms. The arms are always fixed in the same position. (Muscle target group / lower back)

Extended arm to leg lifts

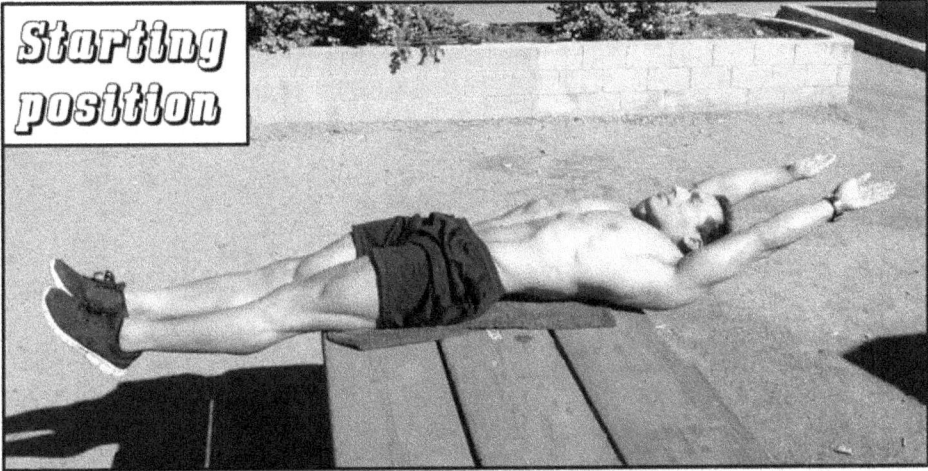

Starting position

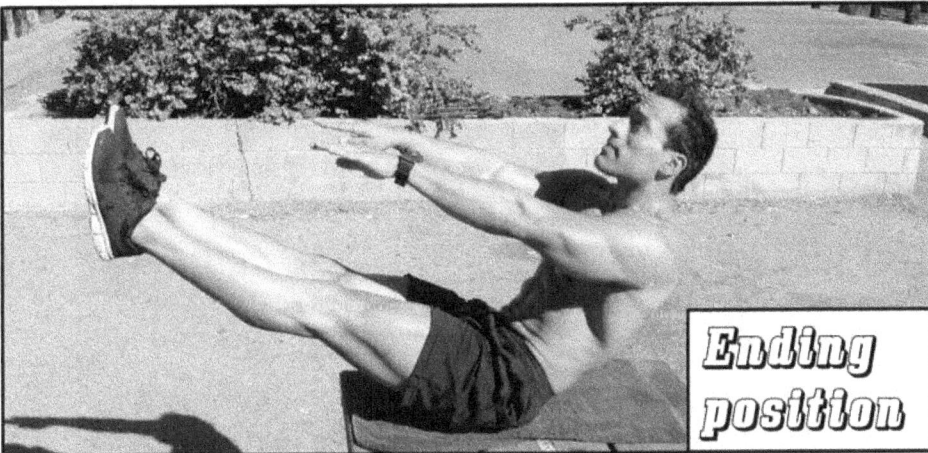

Ending position

1) Lay down on a flat surface extending the legs and arms to a full body stretch.
2) On the exhale, lift the legs and reach forward with the arms towards the toes.
(Muscle target / abbs)

Leg lifts

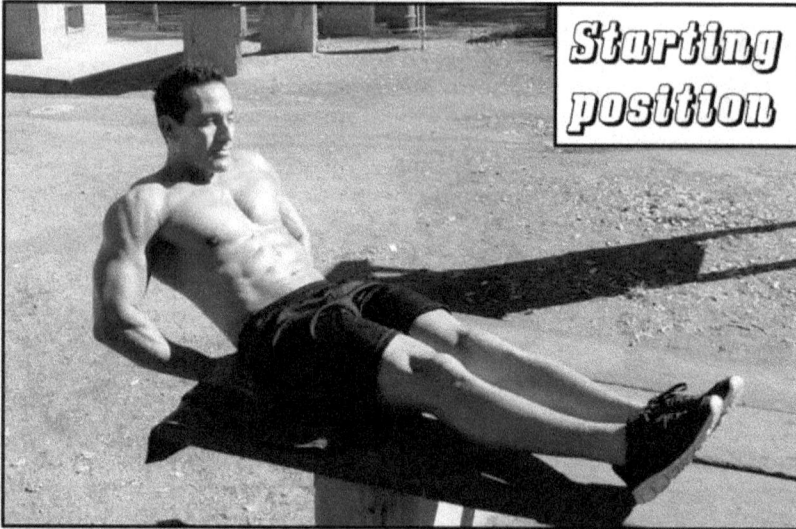

Starting position

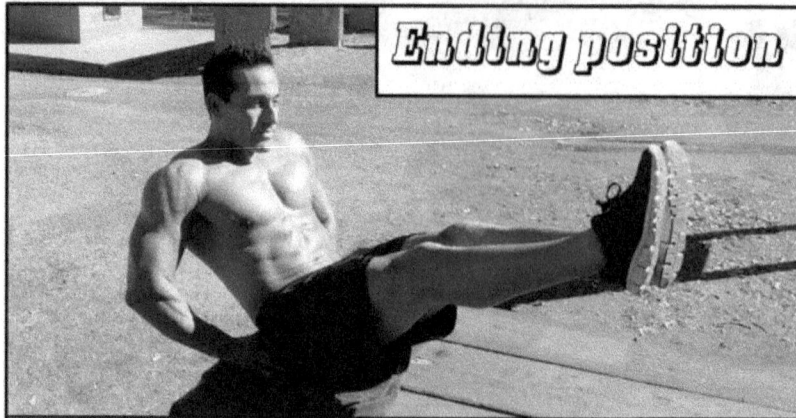

Ending position

1) Sit down on a flat surface and slightly lean back with the legs extended forward.
2) On the exhale, lift the extended legs up.
3) On the inhale, lower the legs back down.
(Muscle target / abbs)

Table crunches

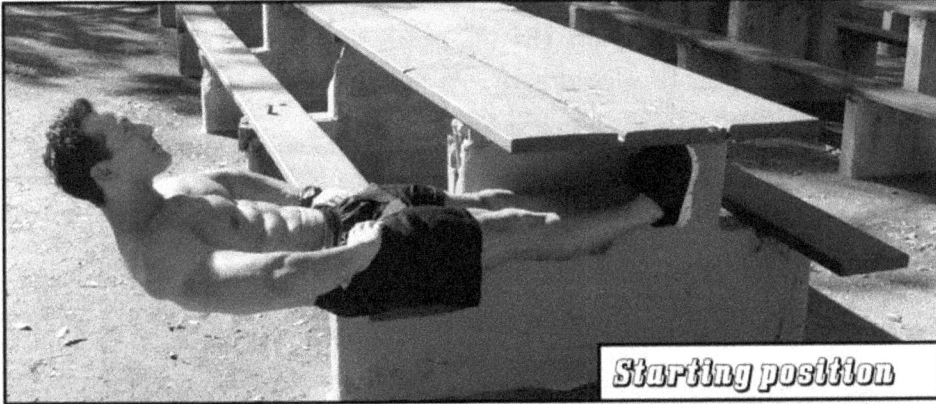

Starting position

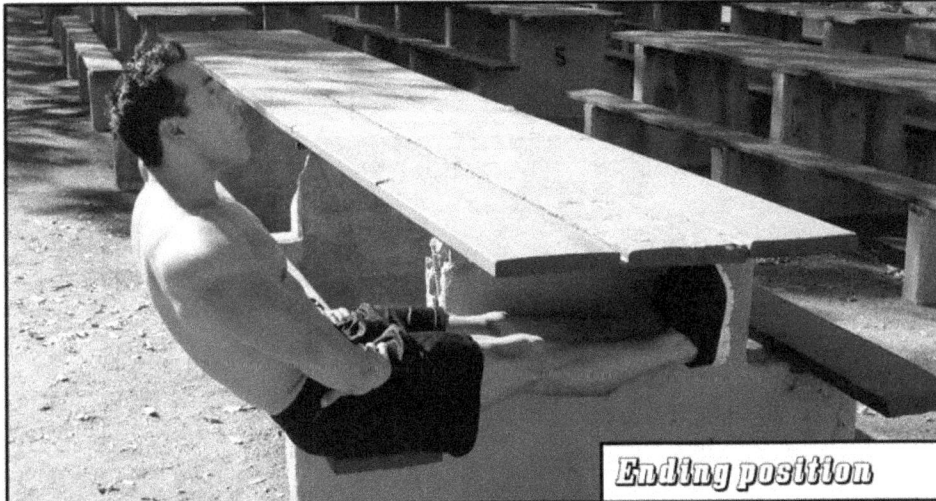

Ending position

1) Keep the legs locked out with the toes firmly planted upward under the table top.
2) On the exhale, crunch up and hold the crunched position for a split second before coming back to the starting position.
3) Inhale on the way down.
(Muscle target / abbs)

Single leg bridge lifts

1) Lay down on a flat surface, extend one leg forward and lift the hips with the other leg.
2) On the exhale, lift the extended leg up. On the inhale, bring the leg down. Do not drop the hips.
(Muscle target / abbs and core)

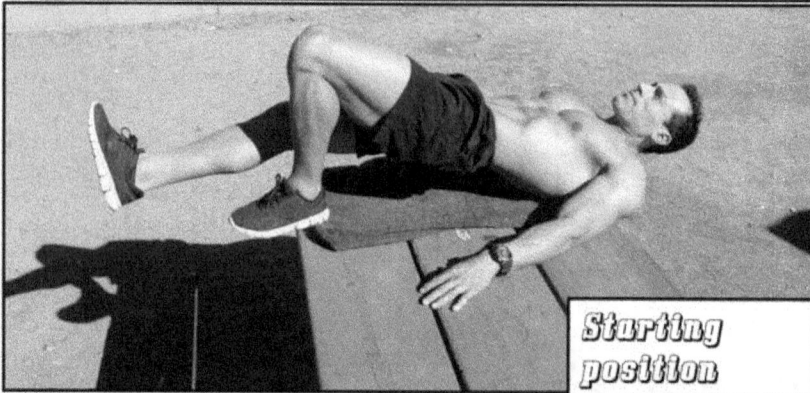

Starting position

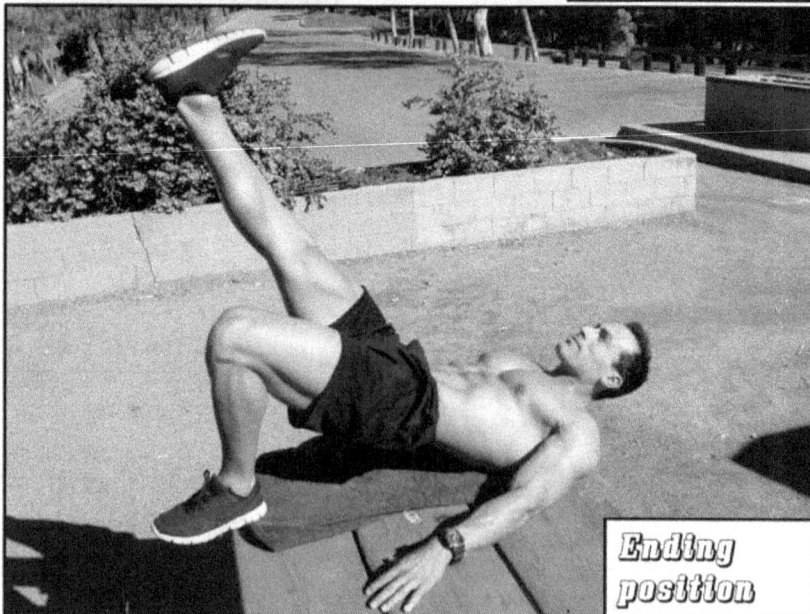

Ending position

Vertical scissors

Neutral position

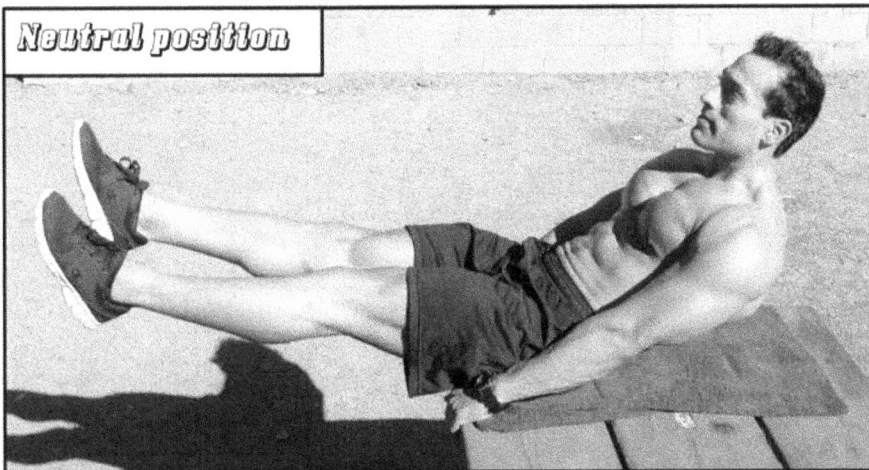

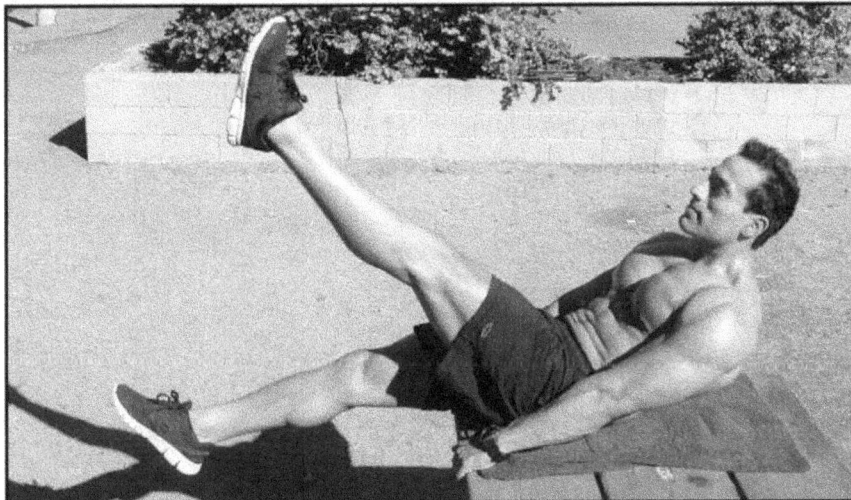

1) Lay down or partially sit down on a flat surface. Keep the hands on the sides and extend the legs forward.
2) Begin to move the legs up and down past each other. Keep the legs straight at all times. (Muscle target / abbs)

Parallel side scissors

Neutral position

1) Lay down or partially sit down on a flat surface. Keep the hands on the sides and extend the legs forward.
2) Begin to move the legs side to side past each other. Keep the legs straight at all times. (Muscle target / abbs)

Plank holds

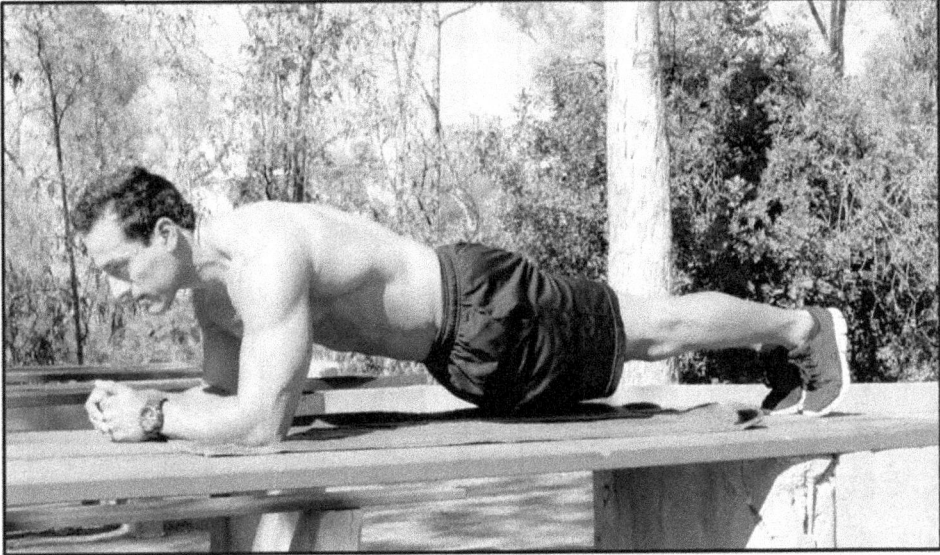

While holding the plank position on a flat surface,
keep the abbs tight. Do not let the mid section
sag. Keep the breathing even and slow.
(Muscle target / abbs and core)

Standing side crunches

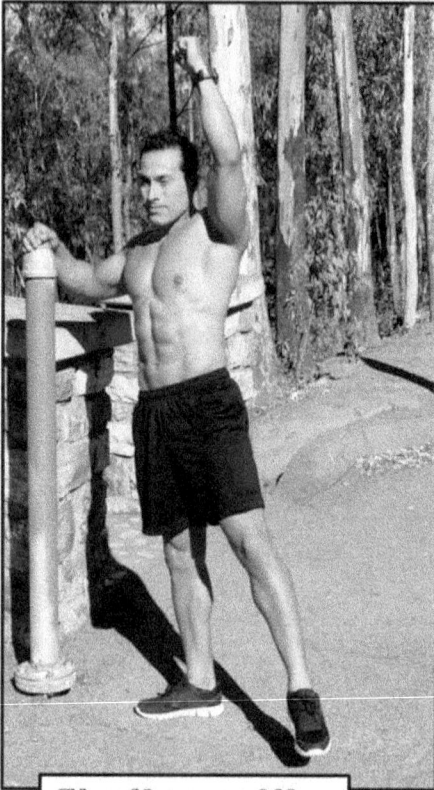

Starting position

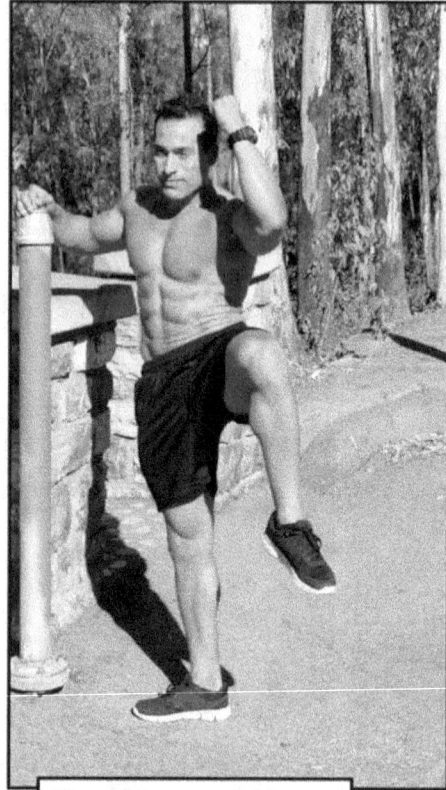

Ending position

1) Place all of the body weight on the back leg, slightly lift the front leg and lift the same side arm as the lifted leg. For balance, it is recommended to hold on to a fixed point.
2) On the exhale, lift and bend the front leg to the side and lower the elbow towards the knee.
(Muscle target /obliques and abbs)

Muay Thai Knee

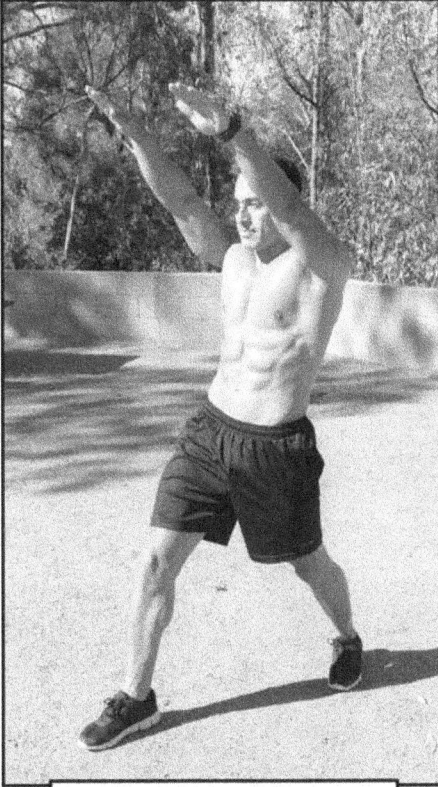

Starting position

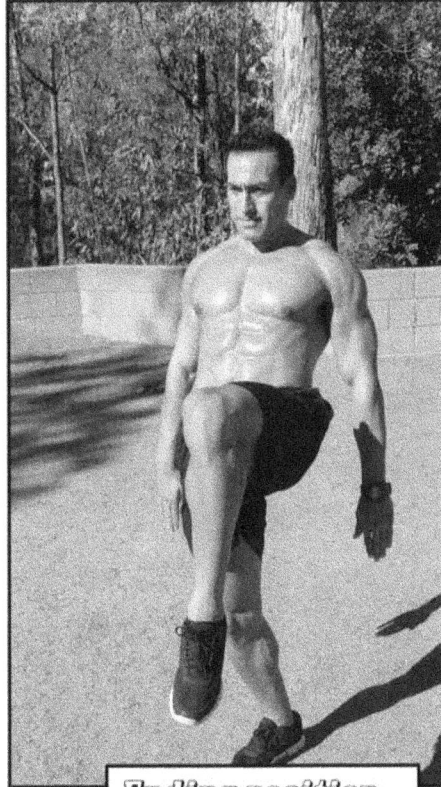

Ending position

1) Start out by standing in a lunge like position with the arms extended forward.
2) On the exhale, lift the back leg forward into a bent knee and tighten the abbs. Bring the arms down to the sides.
(Muscle target / abbs)

Abdominal exhales

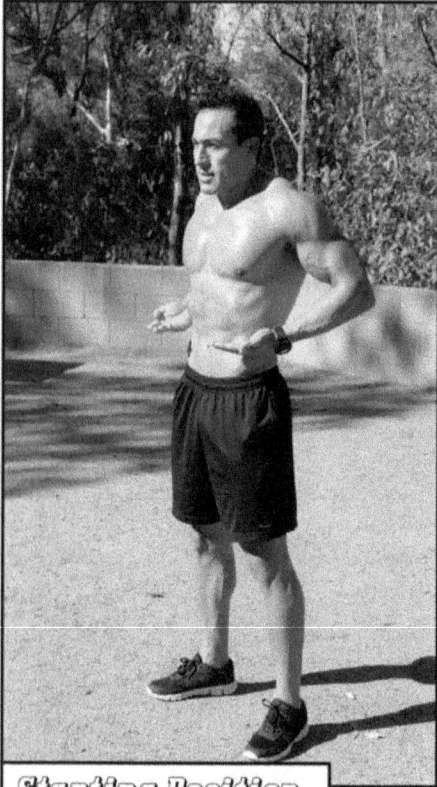

Starting Position

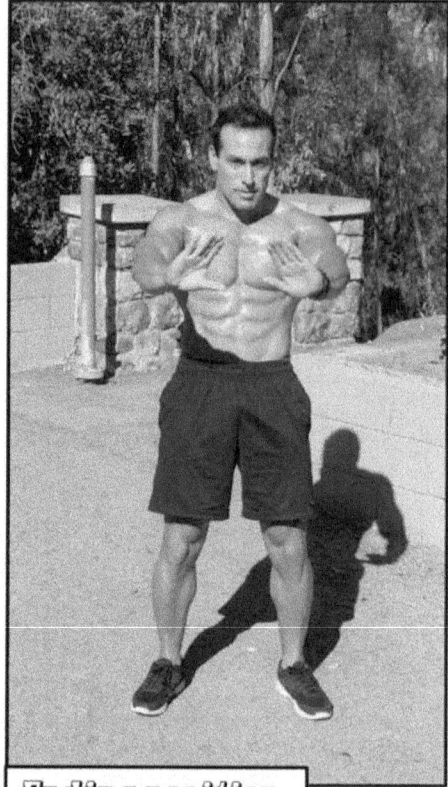

Ending position

1) While standing upright, relax the abbs, inhale and move the elbows back. Keep the palms open and pointing upward.
2) On the exhale contract the abbs, move the arms forward and pause.
(Muscle target / abbs)

Calf raises

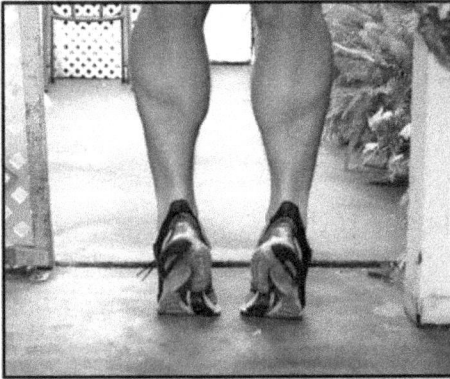

Option 1

Come up on the toes while they are pointing forward. Flex the calves at the top and pause for 3 seconds before taking the heals back to the ground.

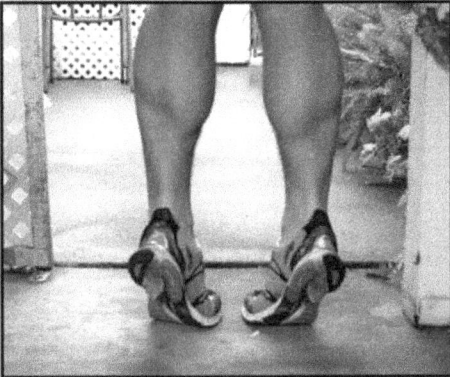

Option 2

Come up on the toes while they are pointing inward. Flex the calves at the top and pause for 3 seconds before taking the heals back to the ground.

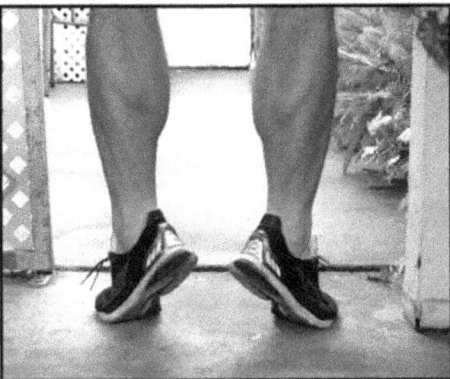

Option 3

Come up on the toes while they are pointing outward. Flex the calves at the top and pause for 3 seconds before taking the heals back to the ground.

CHAPTER 7
THE BASICS WITH WEIGHTS

Two light-moderate weight dumbbells of equal weight should be more than enough for all the exercises presented in this chapter.

How to select the proper dumbbells ?

1. Comfortable grip. If the grip is metal it's a good idea to wear gloves.
2. If you can't functionally perform 15-20 repetitions with reserved strength left after a set, the dumbbells are too heavy.
3. If possible, try to use the type of dumbbell presented in picture A. Not picture B.

Picture A

Solid dumbbells without pointed edges.

Picture B

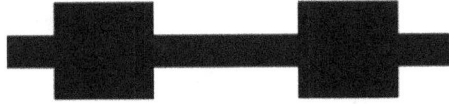

Dumbbells that are not solid have a pointed extending metal handle that sticks out to the sides. This increases the possibility of injury. The use of these dumbbells is not recommended for safety purposes.

Derek Trudeau

Dumbbell press

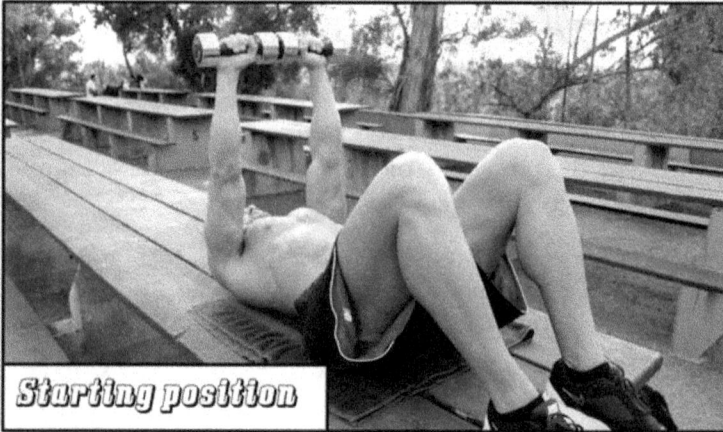

Starting position

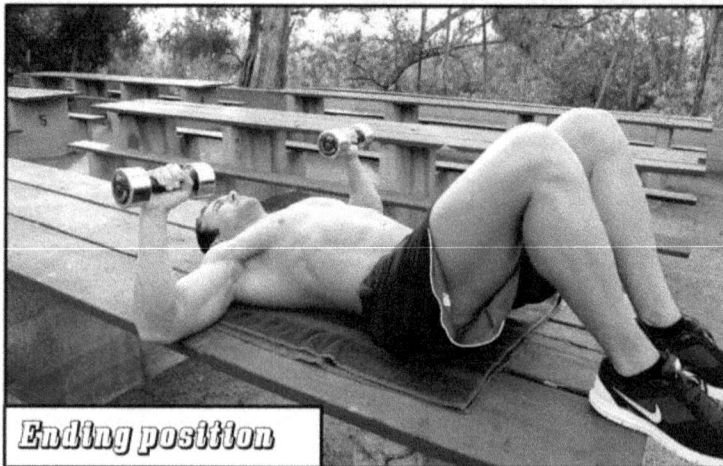

Ending position

Lay down on a flat surface with two dumbbells extended over the chest.
(Have the sides of the dumbbells touching).
1) On the inhale, slowly bring the dumbbells down.
Allow the back of the arms to make contact with the flat surface.
2) On the exhale, lift the dumbbells back up to the starting position and flex
the chest.
(Muscle target / middle chest)

Dumbbell flys

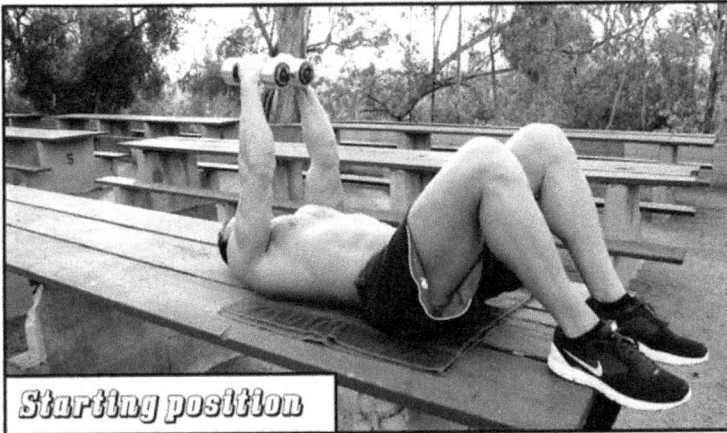

Starting position

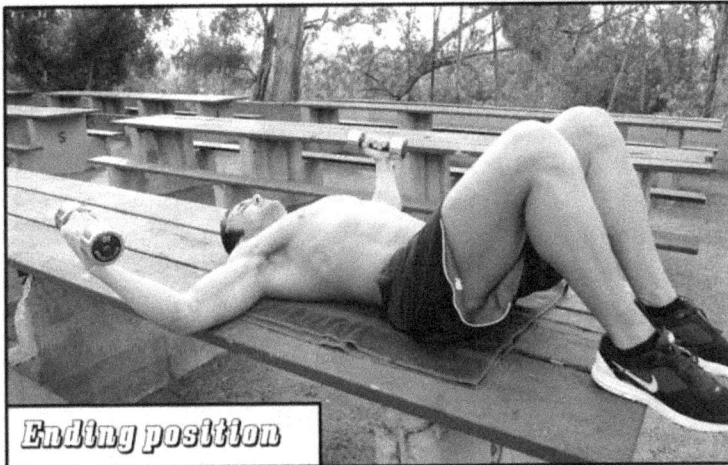

Ending position

Lay down on a flat surface with two dumbbells extended over the chest.
   (Keep the dumbbells parallel to each other).
1) On the inhale, slowly bring the dumbbells down towards the flat surface.
   (Allow for a slight bending to happen at the elbows).
2) On the exhale, fly the dumbbells back up as if you are hugging a tree and
   flex the chest.
(Muscle target / middle chest)

Dumbbell turns

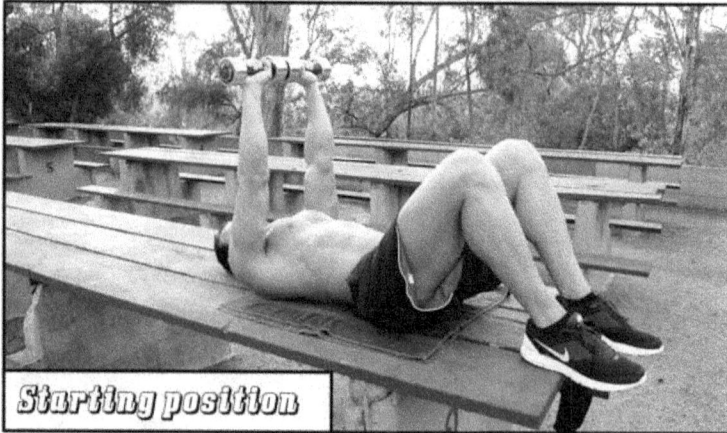
Starting position

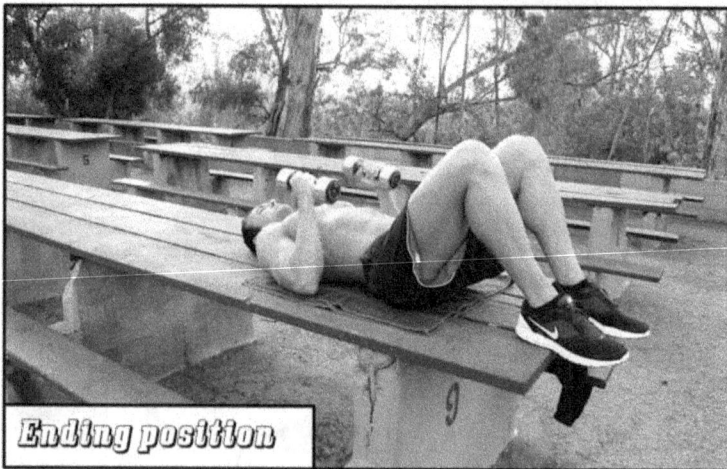
Ending position

Lay down on a flat surface with two dumbbells extended over the chest. (Have the sides of the dumbbells touching).
1) On the inhale, slowly rotate and bring the dumbbells down. (Slide the elbows slowly along the rib cage).
2) On the exhale, lift and turn the dumbbells back to the starting position.
(Muscle target / middle chest)

Incline dumbbell press

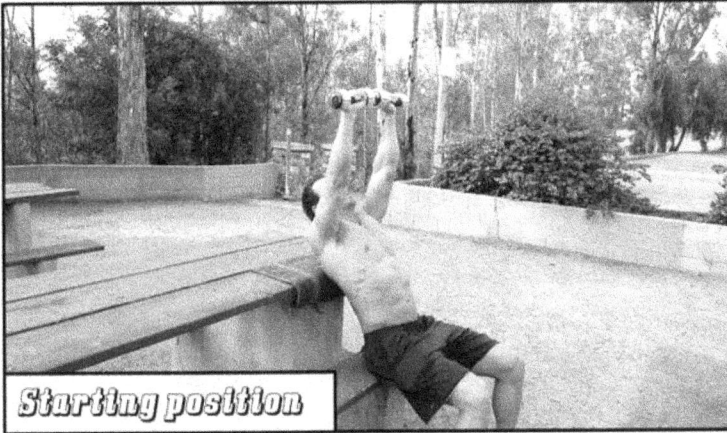

Starting position

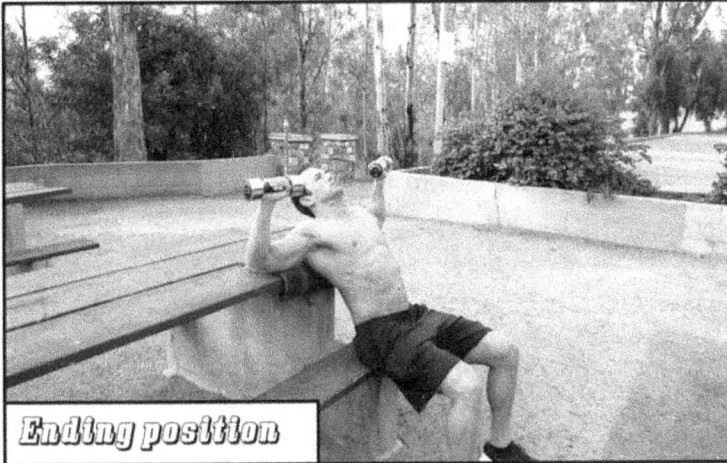

Ending position

Lean on an incline angled surface (a table or a rail works best) with two dumbbells extended over the chest. (Have the sides of the dumbbells touching).
1) On the inhale, slowly bring the dumbbells down towards the shoulders.
2) On the exhale, lift the dumbbells back up to the starting position and flex the chest.
(Muscle target / upper chest)

Incline dumbbell flys

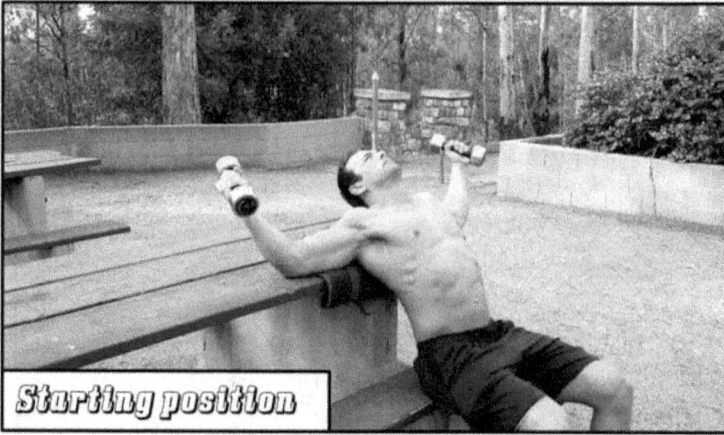

Starting position

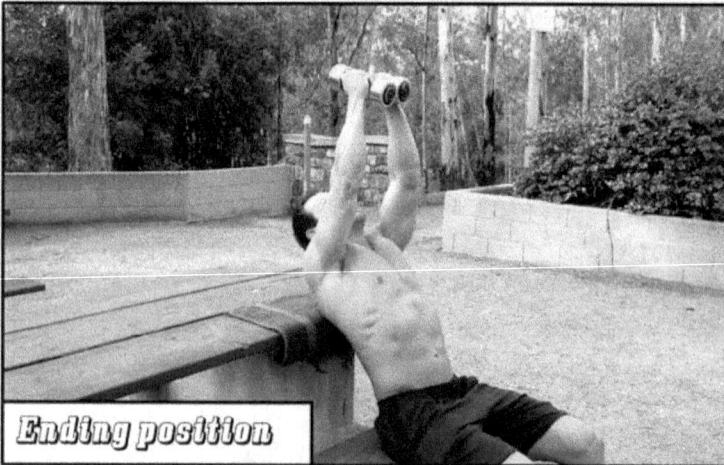

Ending position

Lean on an incline angled surface (a table or a rail works best) with two dumbbells extended over the chest. (Hold the dumbbells parallel to each other).

1) On the inhale, slowly bring the dumbbells down and slightly pop the chest up. (Allow for a slight bending to happen at the elbows).

2) On the exhale, fly the dumbbells back up as if you are hugging a tree and flex the chest.

(Muscle target / upper chest)

Turning dumbbell rows

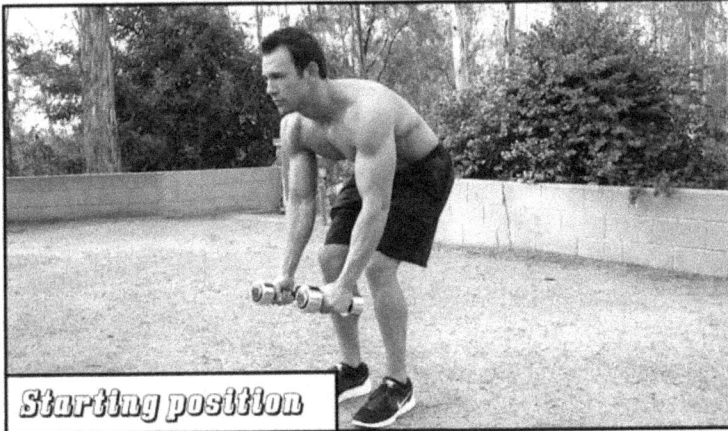

Starting position

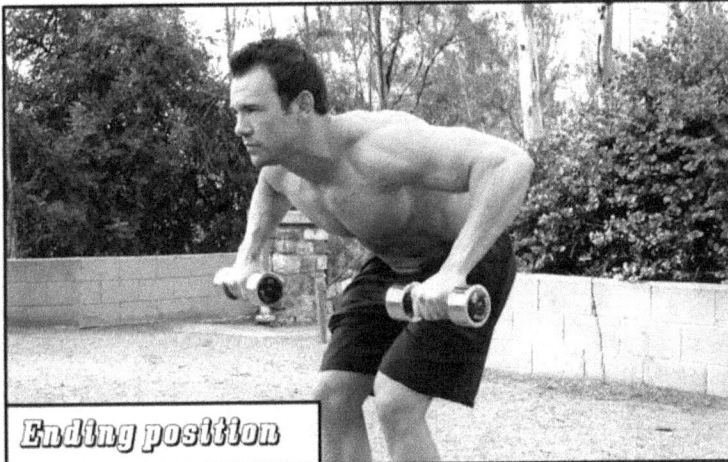

Ending position

Bend the knees and lean forward with the dumbbells positioned parallel to
      each other. (Do not round the back).
1) On the exhale, lift and turn the dumbbells.
2) On the inhale, come back to the starting position.
(Muscle target / lats)

Underhand dumbbell rows

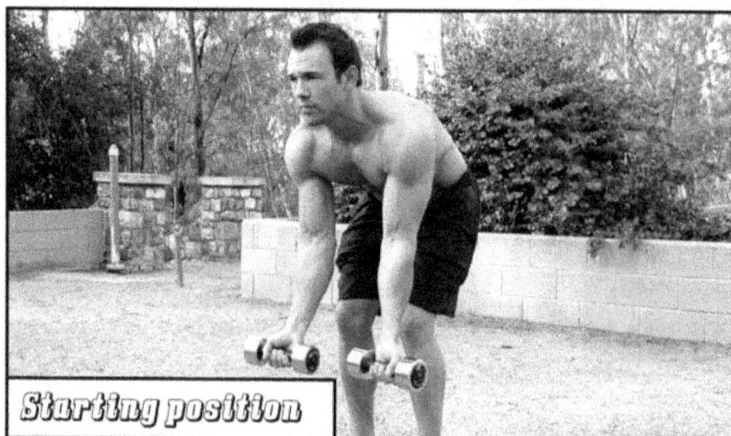

Starting position

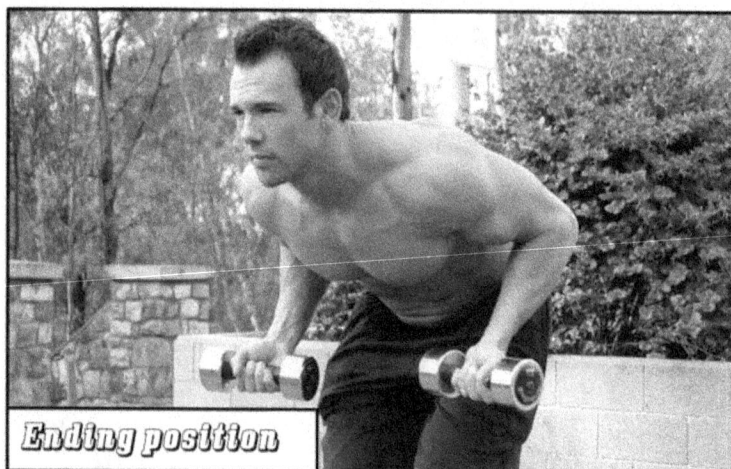

Ending position

Bend the knees and lean forward with the dumbbells at full arm extension. (Hold the dumbbells with an underhand grip).
1) On the exhale, lift the dumbbells up. (Slide the elbows along the rib cage and bring the shoulder blades together).
2) On the inhale, take the dumbbells back down to the starting position. (Do not round the back).
   (Muscle target / lats and biceps)

Wide dumbbell rows

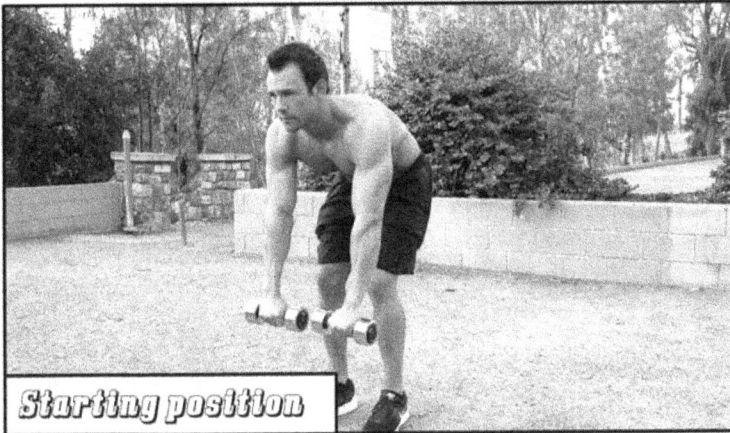

Starting position

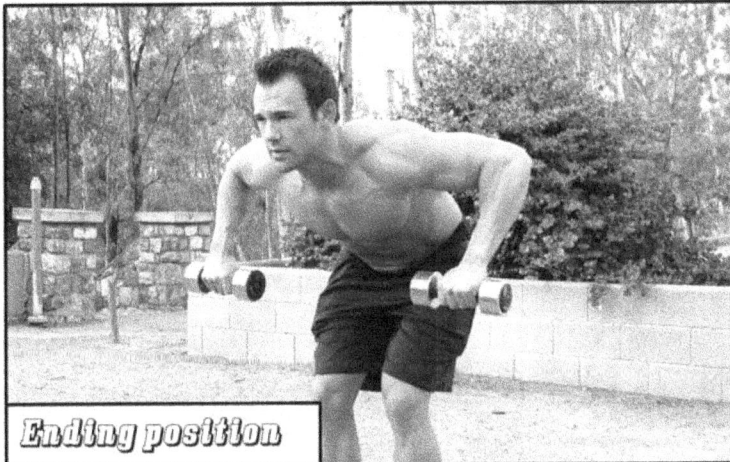

Ending position

Bend the knees and lean forward with the dumbbells at full arm extension. (Do not round the back).
1) On the exhale, lift dumbbells up. (Bring the shoulder blades together).
2) On the inhale, take the dumbbells back to the starting position.
(Muscle target / lats and biceps)

Dumbbell deadlifts

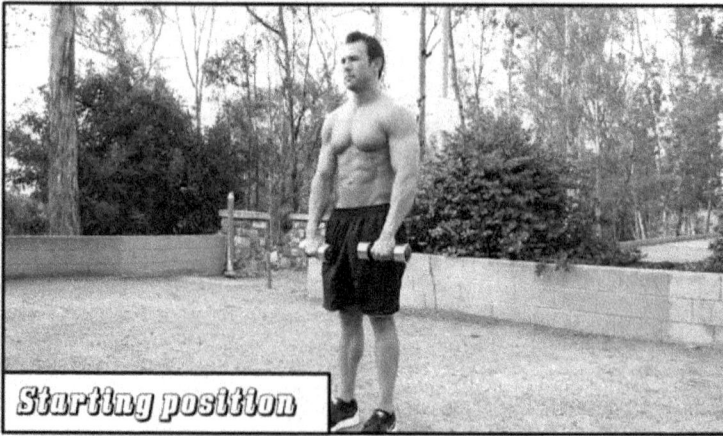
Starting position

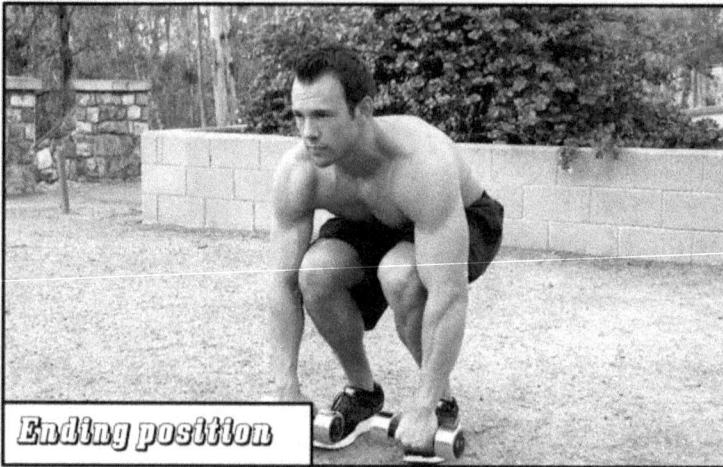
Ending position

1) On the inhale, bend the knees and lean forward with the dumbbells almost touching the ground.
2) On the exhale, come up to the starting position and flex the lower back muscles.
(Muscle target / lower back and legs)

Single dumbbell rows

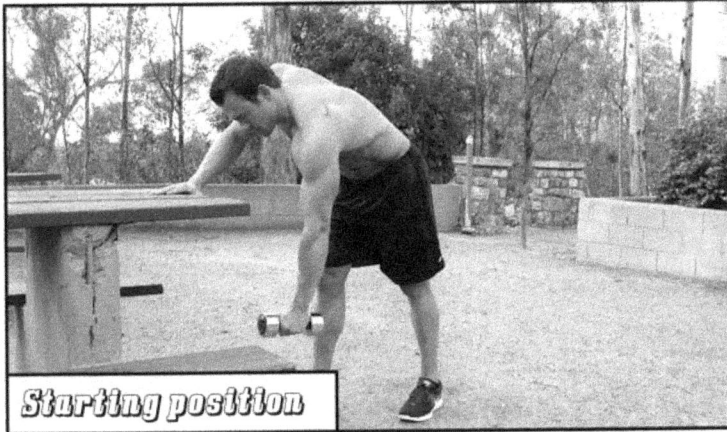

Starting position

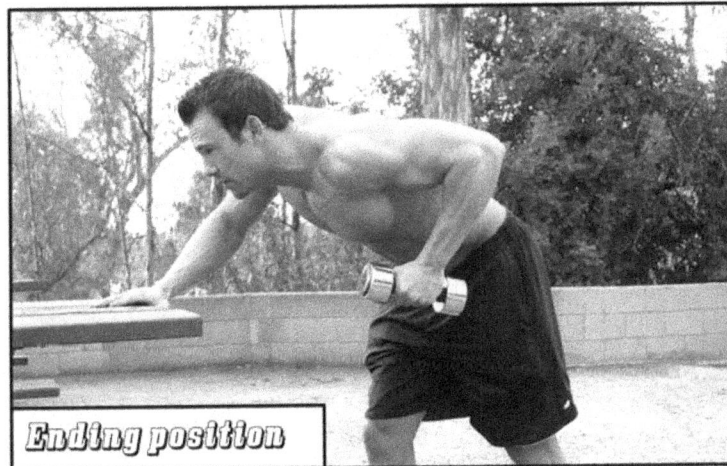

Ending position

Lean forward on a firm platform with one arm while holding a dumbbell in the other arm at full extension.

1) On the exhale, lift the dumbbell up. Slide the elbow along the side of the rib cage.

2) On the inhale, take the dumbbell back down and fully stretch the lat before starting the next repetition.

(Muscle target / lats)

Dumbbell lunges

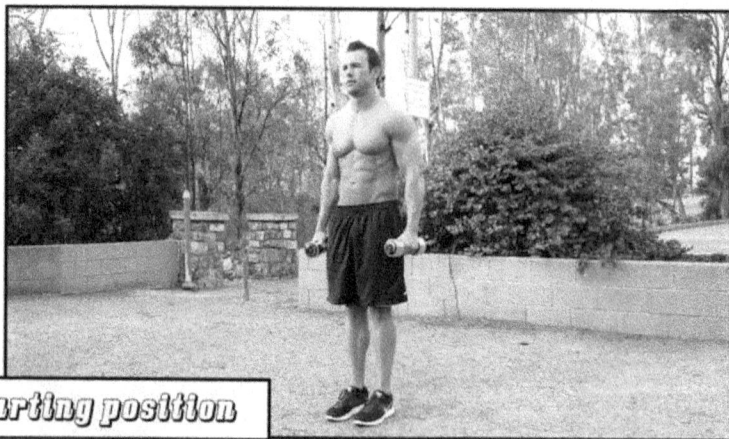

Starting position

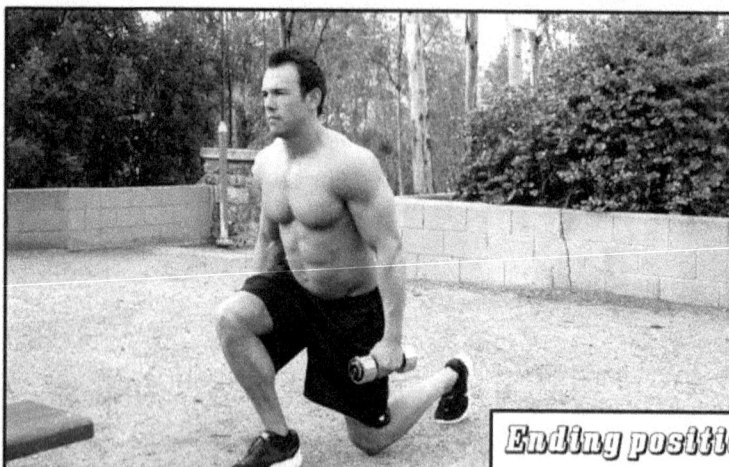

Ending position

1) While holding two dumbbells on the sides, lunge forward with on leg on the inhale.
2) On the exhale, come back to the starting position. (Push off with the heal and try to keep the upper body straight).

(Muscle target / glutes, hams and quads)

Parallel dumbbell squats

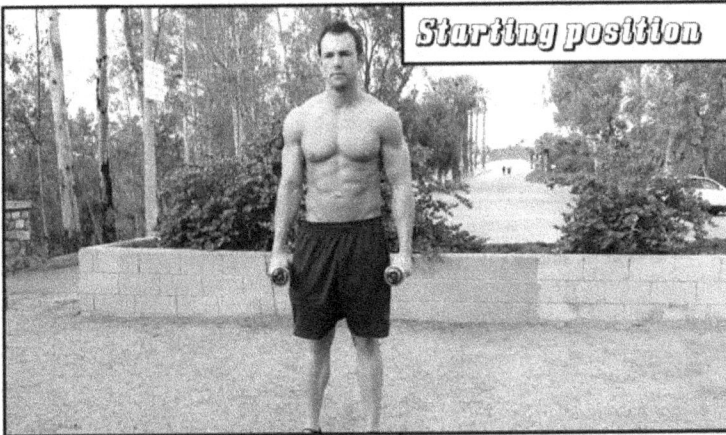

Starting position

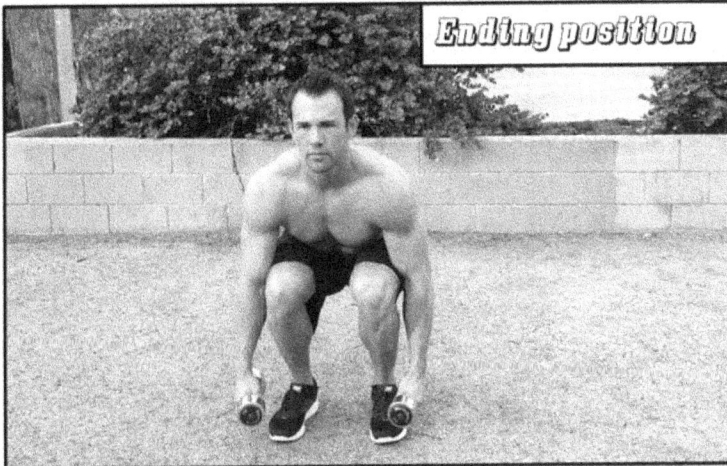

Ending position

Stand straight with dumbbells on the sides.
1) On the inhale, squat down to about 90 degrees.
2) On the exhale, come back up to the starting position and
flex the legs.
(Muscle target / quads)

Sumo dumbbell squats

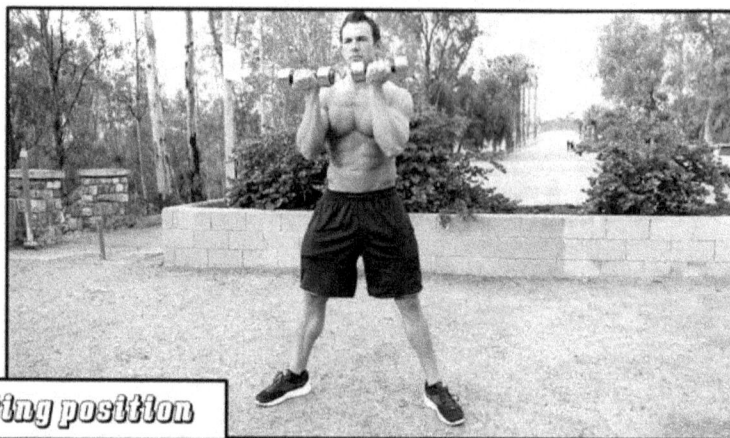

Starting position

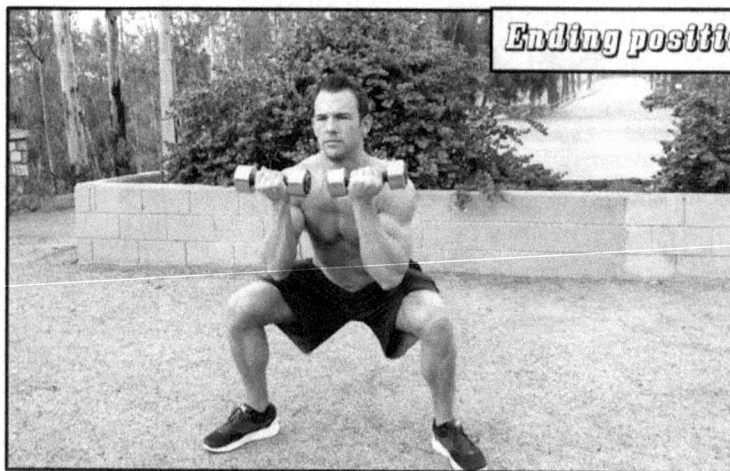

Ending position

Stand straight with the legs wide apart. Keep the toes pointing out and hold the dumbbells by the chest.
1) On the inhale, squat down.
2) On the exhale, come back up.
   (Muscle target / glutes, hams and quads)

Straight leg dumbbell deadlifts

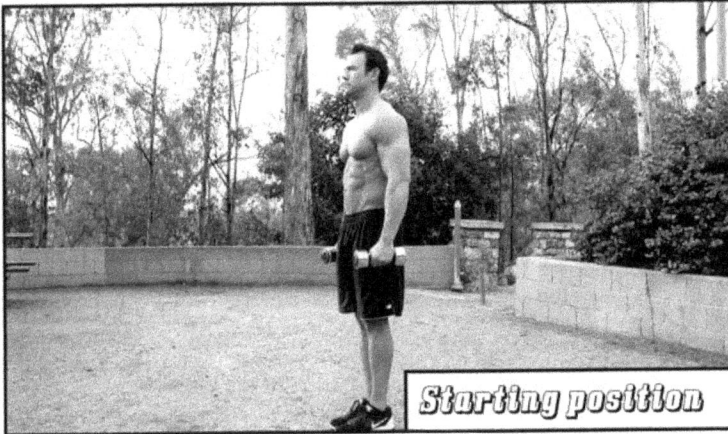

Starting position

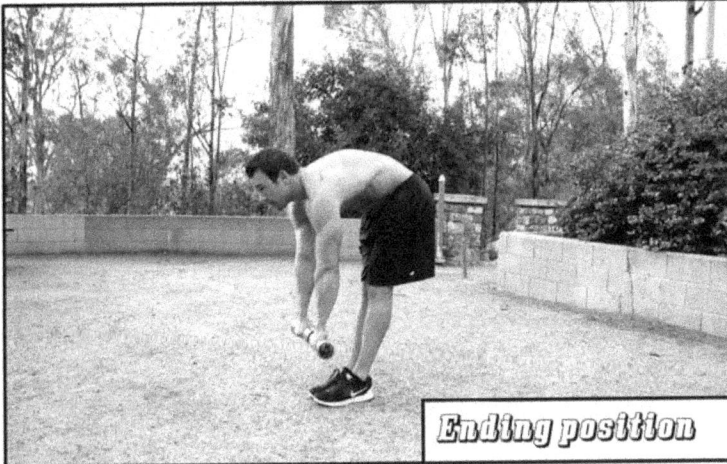

Ending position

Stand straight with the dumbbells in the front or on the sides at full arm extension.
1) On the inhale, slowly take the dumbbells down towards the ground. (Keep the legs locked out).
2) On the exhale, come back up and flex the glutes.
(Muscle target / hams and glutes)

Dumbbell hammer curls

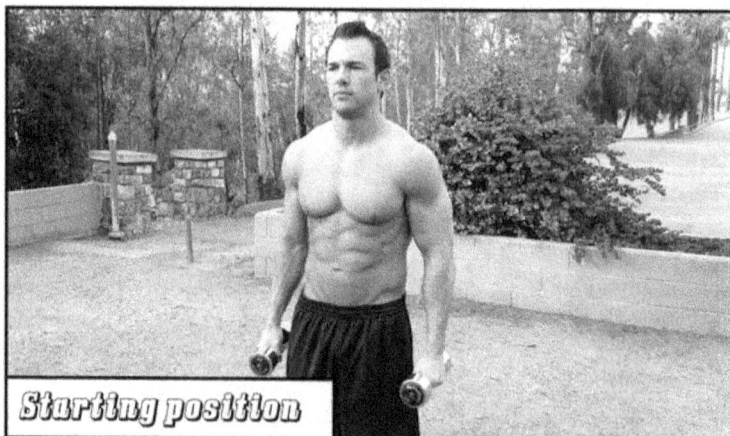

Starting position

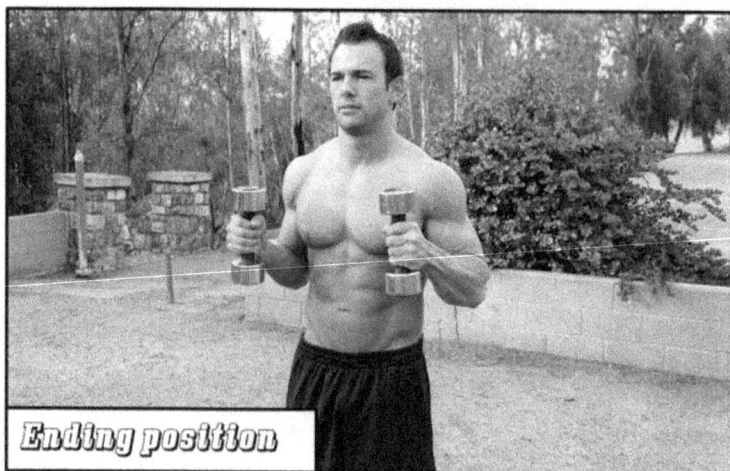

Ending position

Stand straight with the legs slightly bent and the dumbbells on the sides at full arm extension. (Have the dumbbell heads pointing forward).
1) On the exhale, lift the dumbbells up to about 90 degrees and pause for a second before taking the weights back down. (Do not throw the shoulders into the exercise to aid in the lift).
2) On the inhale, take the dumbbells back down to full arm extension. (Muscle target / biceps and forearms)

Dumbbell curls

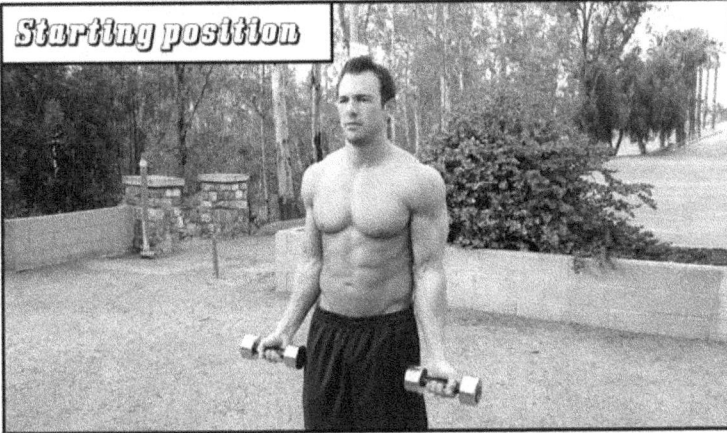

Starting position

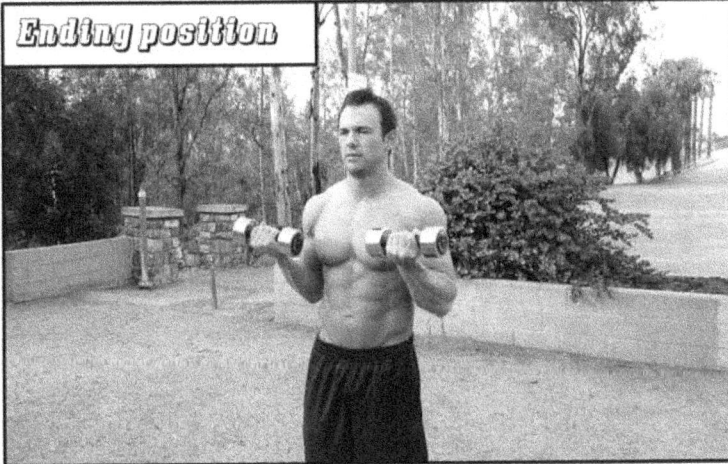

Ending position

Stand straight with the legs slightly bent and the dumbbells on the sides at full arm extension.
1) On the exhale, lift the dumbbells up to shoulder height and pause for a second before taking the weights back down. (Do not throw the shoulders into the exercise to aid in the lift).
2) On the inhale, take the dumbbells back down to full arm extension. (Muscle target / biceps)

Turned out dumbbell curls

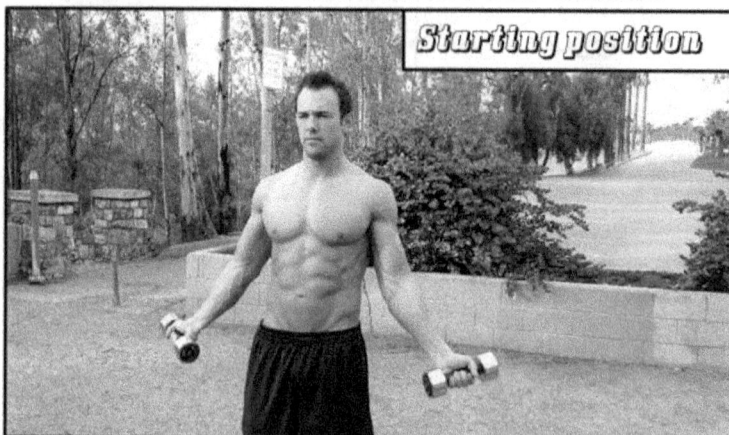

Starting position

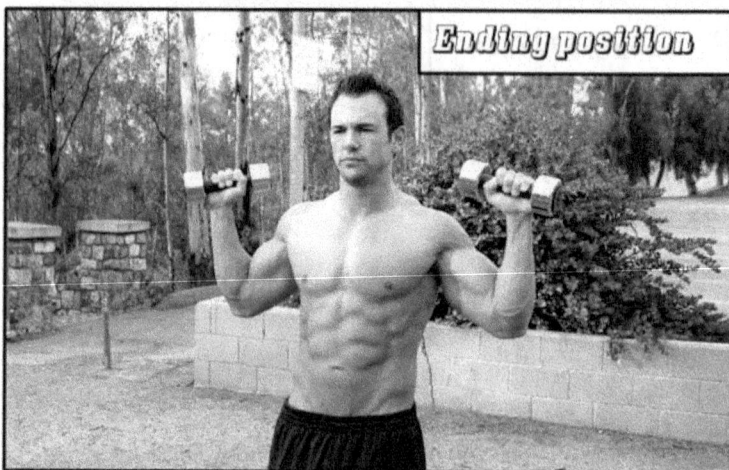

Ending position

Stand straight with the legs slightly bent and the dumbbells on the sides. (Have the dumbbell rotated out so that the thumbs are pointing away from the body).
1) On the exhale, lift the dumbbells over the shoulders and pause for a second before taking the weights back down.
2) On the inhale, take the dumbbells back down to full arm extension.
(Muscle target / biceps and forearms)

Dumbbell kickbacks

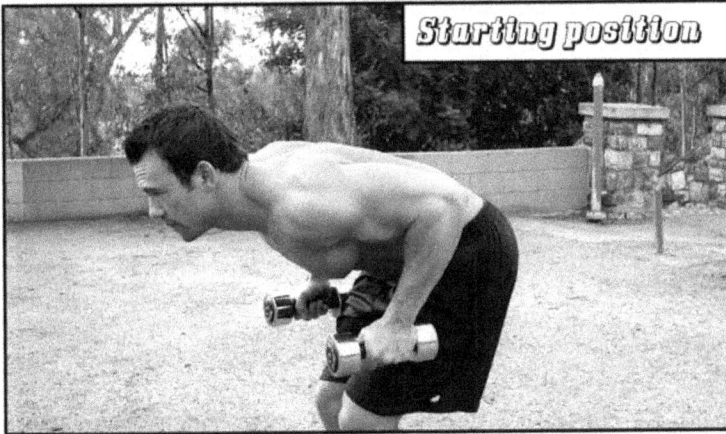

Starting position

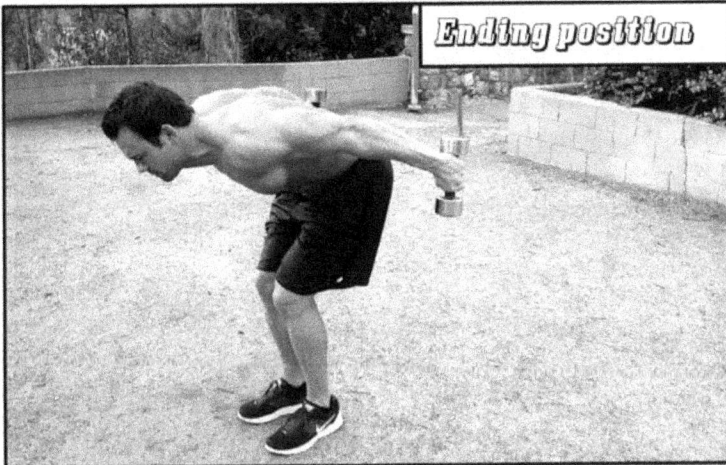

Ending position

Bend the knees and lean forward with the elbows pulled back.
1) On the exhale, lift the dumbbells in reverse. (Do not drop the elbows when lifting the dumbbells back).
2) On the inhale, take the dumbbells back to the starting position.
(Muscle target / triceps)

Dumbbell lateral raises

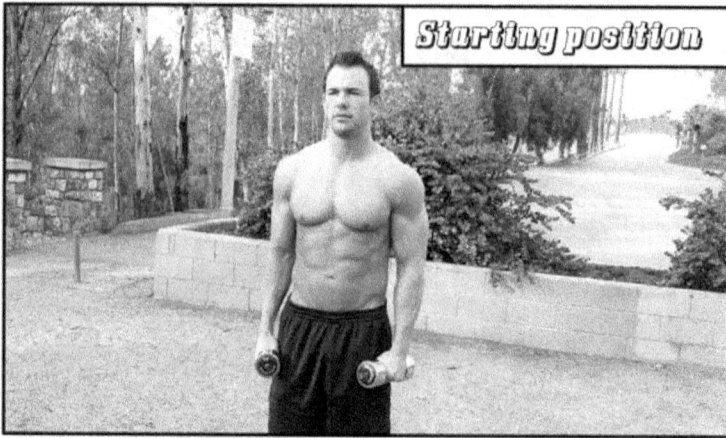

Starting position

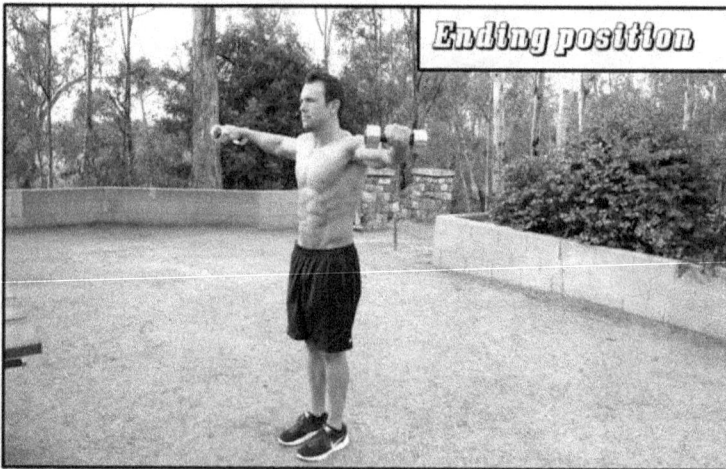

Ending position

Stand straight with the knees slightly bent. (Hold the dumbbells on the sides).
1) On the exhale, lift the dumbbells up towards a parallel with the ground position. (Keep the bending of the elbows at a minimum).
2) On the inhale, take the dumbbells back to the starting position. (Muscle target / deltoids)

Rear dumbbell lateral raises

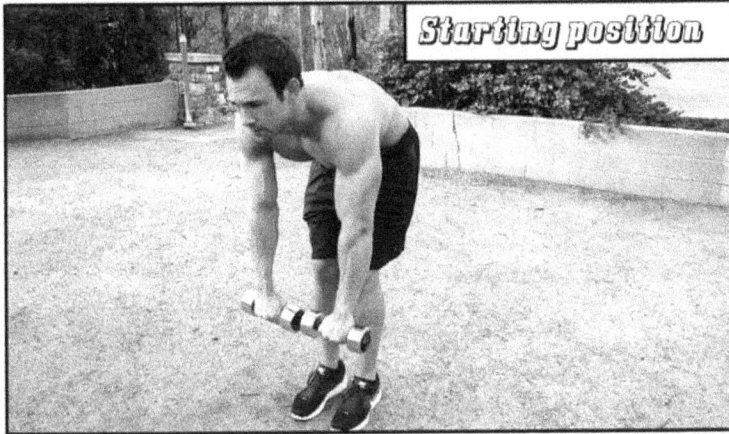

Starting position

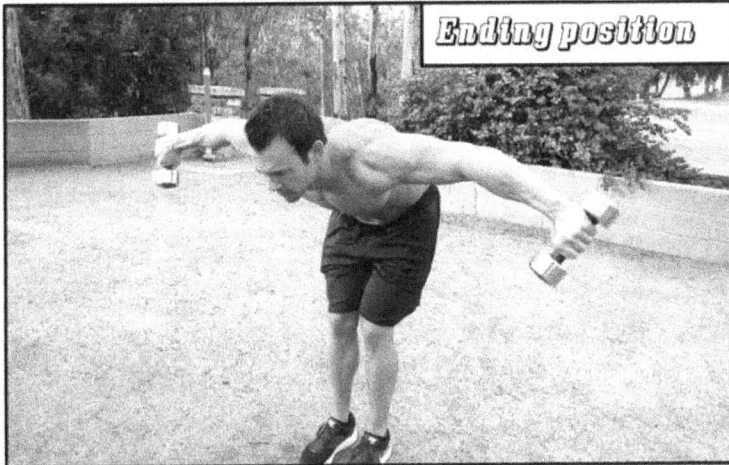

Ending position

Lean forward with the knees bent. (Hold the dumbbells in the front. Do not round the back).
1) On the exhale, lift the dumbbells up towards a parallel with the ground position. (Point the thumbs towards each other when holding the dumbbells).
2) On the inhale, take the dumbbells back to the starting position. (Muscle target / rear deltoids)

Front dumbbell raises

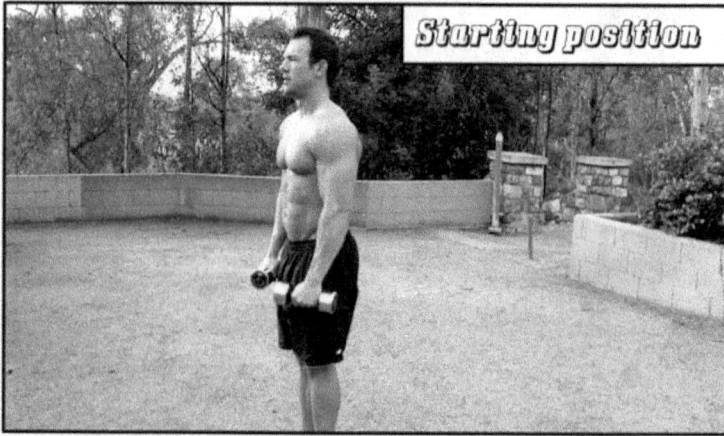

Starting position

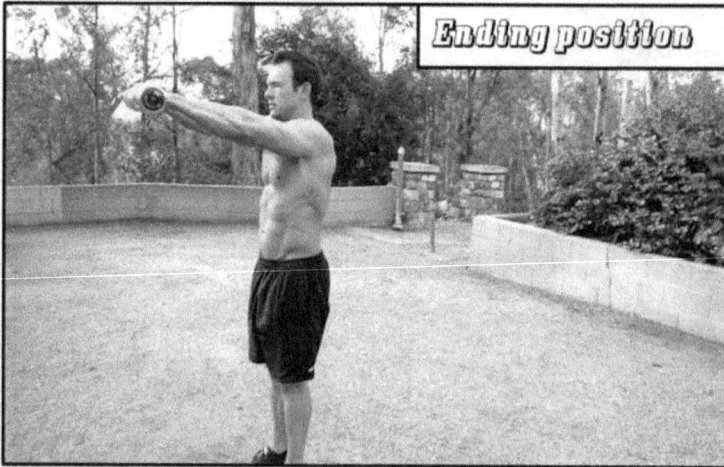

Ending position

Stand straight with the knees slightly bent. (Hold the dumbbells in the front at full arm extension. Have the thumbs pointing towards each other).

1) On the exhale, lift the dumbbells up towards a parallel with the ground position. (Pause for a second at the top before taking the dumbbells back down. keep the arms straight at all times).

2) On the inhale, bring the dumbbells back to the starting position.

Flipped dumbbell shrugs

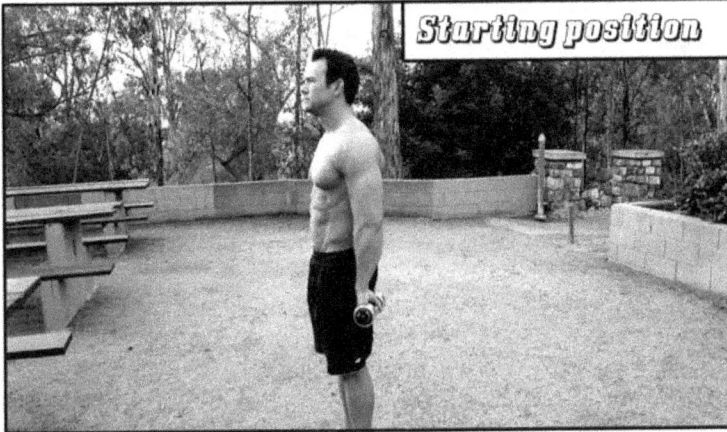

Starting position

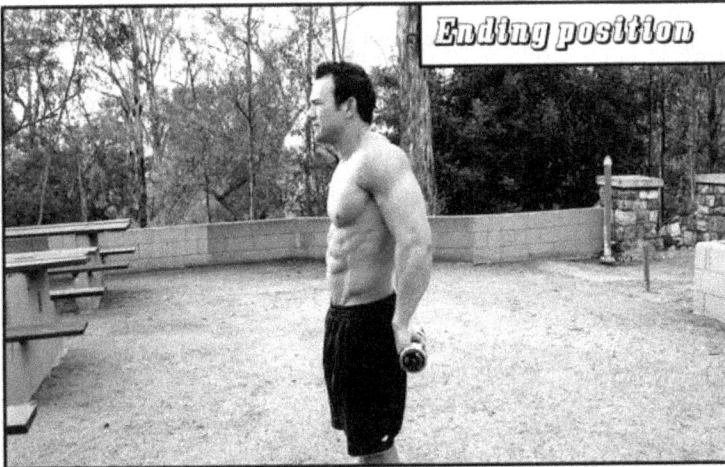

Ending position

Stand straight with the knees slightly bent. (Hold the dumbbells behind the glutes with a reverse grip. The elbows are to point away from the body).
1) On the exhale, lift the dumbbells up with the traps. Pretend that you are trying to touch the ears with the shoulders.
2) Pause at the top and contract the traps for 3 seconds before taking the dumbbells back down to a full stretch. (Only lift with the traps, not the arms).
3) On the inhale, slowly lower the dumbbells back to the starting position.
 (Muscle target / traps)

Military dumbbell press

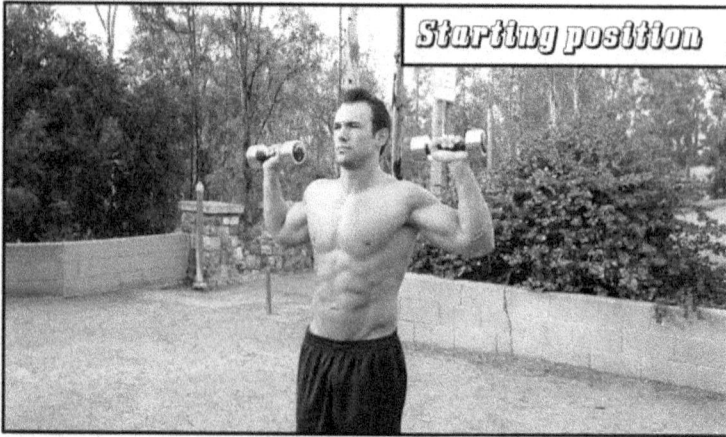
Starting position

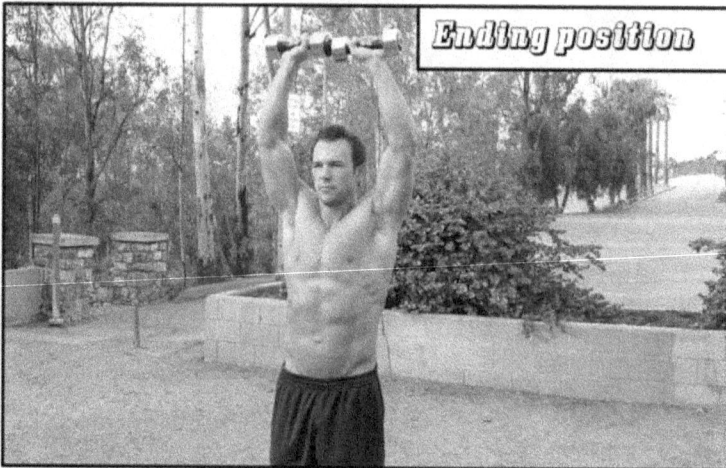
Ending position

Stand straight with the knees slightly bent. (Hold the dumbbells on the sides at or above shoulder height).
1) On the exhale, lift the dumbbells up. (Keep the abbs and the lower back tight at all times. Allow the dumbbells to make contact at the top).
2) On the inhale, slowly take the dumbbells back to the starting position.
(Muscle target / deltoids)

Dumbbell table crunches

Starting position

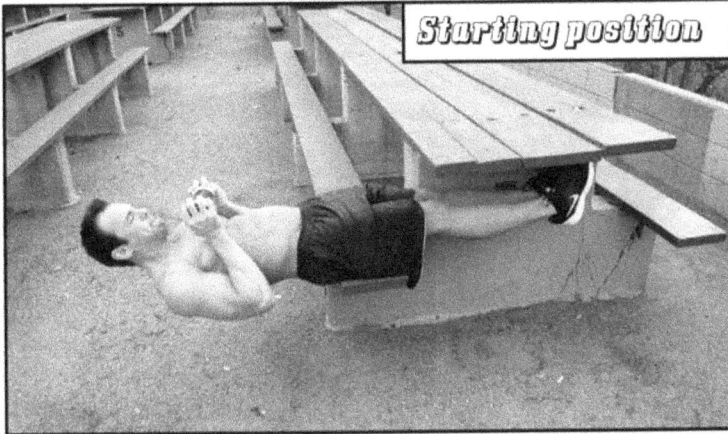

Ending position

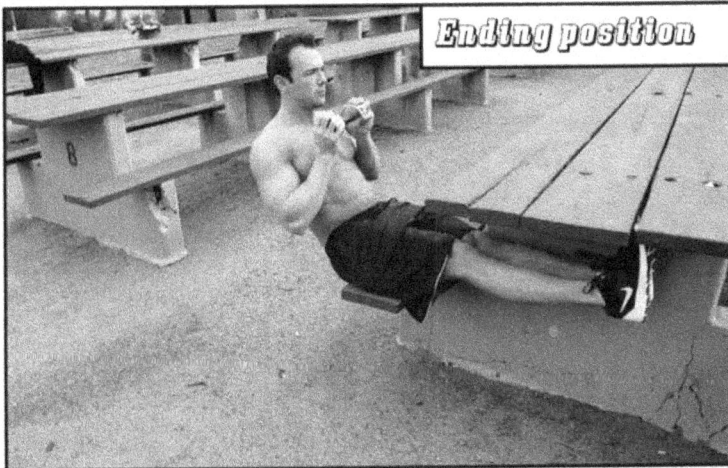

Keep the legs locked out with the toes firmly planted upward under the table top. (Hold a dumbbell with both hands on the chest or behind the head).
1) On the exhale, crunch up and hold the crunched position for a split second before coming back to the starting position. (Inhale on the way down).
(Muscle target / abbs)

Dumbbell chest crunches

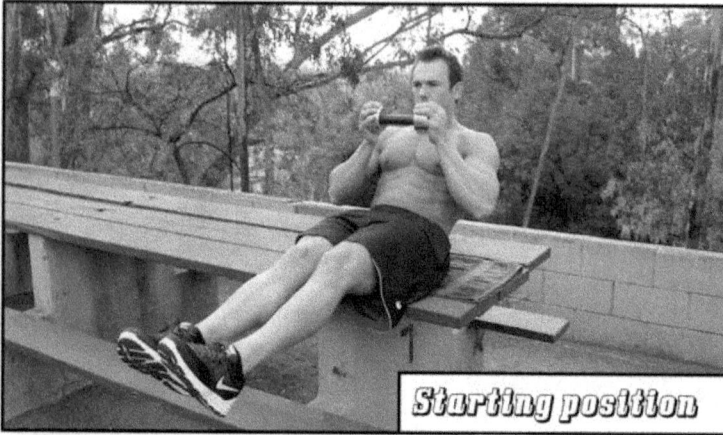

Starting position

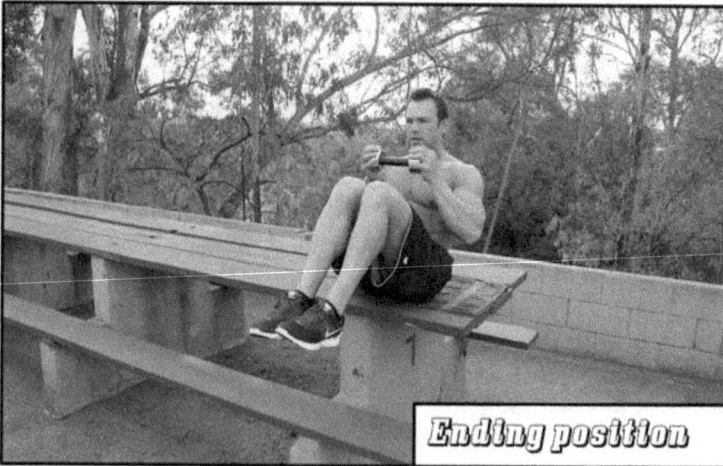

Ending position

Lay down or slightly sit up on a flat surface. (Hold a dumbbell over the chest and extend the legs forward above the ground).
1) On the exhale, crunch up and bend the legs toward the chest.
2) On the inhale, come back to the starting position.

Dumbbell single leg mini crunches

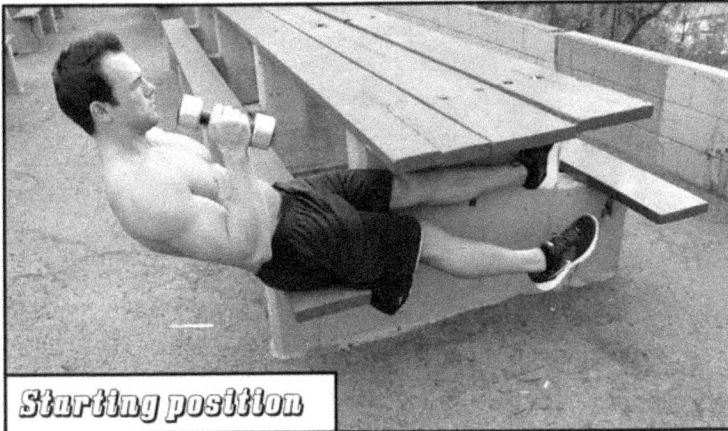

Starting position

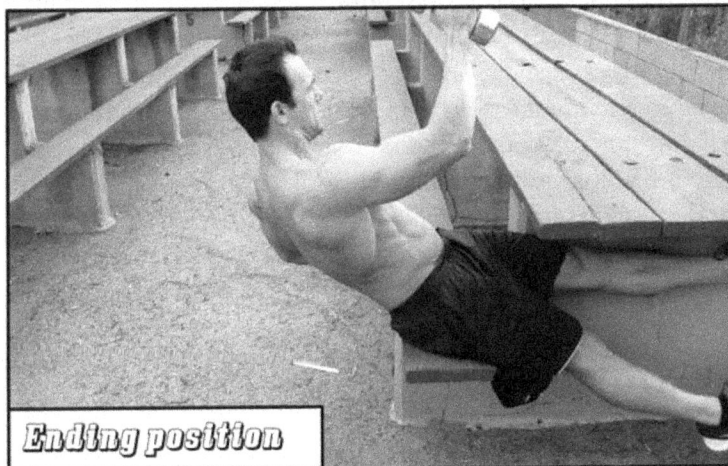

Ending position

Keep one leg locked out with the toes firmly planted upward under the table top. (Hold a dumbbell with an opposite hand).
1) On the exhale, crunch twist up with the dumbbell to the opposite side. (Inhale on the way down).
(Muscle target / abbs)

CHAPTER 8
THE 16 WEEK APPROACH

The 16 week approach can also be viewed as a 16 step process. The rules are clear. **<u>Do Not</u>** move on to the next (week/step) until you can comfortably finish the (week/step) that you are on. It's possible that some individuals will be on a certain week for some time before moving on to the next one. That's normal, do not give up. So what if it takes you longer. No one said it would be easy. Your Hollywood abbs will come if you stay the course. Remember the chapter on the starting point? My fat ass started at 250 lbs and a bad knee. It took me one month to move from step 4 to step 5. But now, as my Hollywood abbs smile back at me in the mirror, I don't care how long it would have taken to move up from step to step. The fight was well worth it in the end.

(Note) Do not cheat! Stay at the step/week you are on until you can comfortably complete it.

(Note) Every week select five days for mandatory training. The other two days may be utilized for rest or as (cardio and abb days). Cheating and skipping training steps goes against Hollywood abbs commandments # 1, 9 and 10.

(Note) Remember the sixth Hollywood abbs commandment.
If the body hurts, rest and recover. But always maintain a clean diet.

Week 1 Cardio	Training routine

Day1
 	
Slow jog 1 mile
	Chest and Abbs
	1. Standard pushups/ 3 sets of 10 (or) hold the pushup position 3 times. Once the burn starts, count down from 10 then stop. **(pg 45)**
	2. Wide pushups/ 3 sets of 10 (or) hold the wide pushup position 3 times as long as possible. **(pg 46)**
	3. Dumbbell press/ 3 sets of 10 **(pg 64)**
	4. Dumbbell flys/ 3 sets of 10 **(pg 65)**
	5. Dumbbell turns/ 3 sets of 10 **(pg 66)**
	(Abbs) --
	   • Vertical scissors / 3 sets of 10 **(pg 55)**
	   • Single leg bridge lifts/ 3 sets of 10 (each side) **(pg 54)**
	   • Parallel side scissors/ 3 sets of 10 **(pg 56)**

Day2
 	
Slow jog 1 mile
	Back and Abbs
	1. Underhand bar pulls/ 3 sets of 10 or hold the contracted position at the top 3 times. Once the burn starts, count down from 10 then stop. **(pg 44)**
	2. Turning dumbbell rows/ 3 sets of 10 **(pg 69)**
	3. Underhand dumbbell rows/ 3 sets of 10 **(pg 70)**
	4. Standing lower back extensions/ 3 sets of 10 **(pg 50)**
	5. Single dumbbell rows / 3 sets of 10 (each side) **(pg 73)**
	(Abbs) --
	   • Vertical scissors / 3 sets of 10 **(pg 55)**
	   • Single leg bridge lifts/ 3 sets of 10 (each side) **(pg 54)**
	   • Parallel side scissors/ 3 sets of 10 **(pg 56)**
	   • Table crunches/ 3 sets of 10 **(pg 53)**

Day3
 	
Slow jog 1 mile
	Legs and Abbs
	1. Parallel close squats/ 3 sets of 10 **(pg 49)**
	2. Sumo squats/ 3 sets of 10 **(pg 48)**
	3. Dumbbell lunges/ 3 sets of 10 **(pg 74)**
	4. Straight leg dumbbell deadlifts/ 3 sets of 10 **(pg 77)**
	5. Sumo dumbbell squats/ 3 sets of 10 **(pg 76)**
	(Abbs) --
	   • Vertical scissors / 3 sets of 10 **(pg 55)**
	   • Single leg bridge lifts/ 3 sets of 10 (each side) **(pg 54)**
	   • Parallel side scissors/ 3 sets of 10 **(pg 56)**
	   • Table crunches/ 3 sets of 10 **(pg 53)**

Week 1

Cardio	Training routine
Day4 Slow jog 1 mile	**Arms and Abbs** 1. Single side wall pulls / 3 sets of 10 (each side) **(pg 42)** 2. Dumbbell hammer curls/ 3 sets of 10 **(pg 78)** 3. Close pushups/ 3 sets of 10 (or) hold the close pushup position 3 times. Once the burn starts, count down from 10 then stop. **(pg 47)** 4. Dumbbell curls/ 3 sets of 10 **(pg 79)** 5. Dumbbell kickbacks/ 3 sets of 10 **(pg 81)** (Abbs) -- • Vertical scissors / 3 sets of 10 **(pg 55)** • Single leg bridge lifts/ 3 sets of 10 (each side) **(pg 54)** • Parallel side scissors/ 3 sets of 10 **(pg 56)** • Table crunches/ 3 sets of 10 **(pg 53)**
Day5 Slow jog 1 mile	**Shoulders and Abbs** 1. Shoulder holds/ 3 times. Once the burn starts, count down from 10 then stop. **(pg 41)** 2. Dumbbell lateral raises/ 3 sets of 10 **(pg 82)** 3. Rear dumbbell raises/ 3 sets of 10 **(pg 83)** 4. Front dumbbell raises/ 3 sets of 10 **(pg 84)** 5. Military dumbbell press/ 3 sets of 10 **(pg 86)** (Abbs) -- • Vertical scissors / 3 sets of 10 **(pg 55)** • Single leg bridge lifts/ 3 sets of 10 (each side) **(pg 54)** • Parallel side scissors/ 3 sets of 10 **(pg 56)** • Table crunches/ 3 sets of 10 **(pg 53)**
Day6 **Optional** 2-3 mile walk	**Abbs** • Choose any 4 abdominal exercises from the book. Perform 4 sets of 10 repetitions per exercise. Be sure to switch sides for exercises that only hit one side of the abdominals at a time.
Day7 **Optional** 2-3 mile walk	**Abbs** • Choose any 4 abdominal exercises from the book. Perform 4 sets of 10 repetitions per exercise. Be sure to switch sides for exercises that only hit one side of the abdominals at a time.

Week 2

Cardio	Training routine
Day1 Slow jog 1.5 miles	**Chest and Abbs** 1. Standard pushups/ 3 sets of 10 (or) hold the pushup position 3 times. Once the burn starts, count down from 10 then stop. **(pg 45)** 2. Wide pushups/ 3 sets of 10 (or) hold the wide pushup position 3 times as long as possible. **(pg 46)** 3. Incline dumbbell press/ 3 sets of 10 **(pg 67)** 4. Incline dumbbell flys/ 3 sets of 10 **(pg 68)** 5. Dumbbell turns/ 3 sets of 10 **(pg 66)** (Abbs) -- • Vertical scissors / 4 sets of 10 **(pg 55)** • Single leg bridge lifts/ 4 sets of 10 (each side) **(pg 54)** • Parallel side scissors/ 4 sets of 10 **(pg 56)**
Day2 Slow jog 1.5 miles	**Back and Abbs** 1. Wide overhand bar pulls/ 3 sets of 10 or hold the contracted position at the top 3 times. Once the burn starts, count down from 10 then stop. **(pg 43)** 2. Turning dumbbell rows/ 3 sets of 10 **(pg 69)** 3. Wide dumbbell rows/ 3 sets of 10 **(pg 71)** 4. Standing lower back extensions/ 3 sets of 10 **(pg 50)** 5. Single dumbbell rows / 3 sets of 10 (each side) **(pg 73)** (Abbs) -- • Vertical scissors / 4 sets of 10 **(pg 55)** • Single leg bridge lifts/ 4 sets of 10 (each side) **(pg 54)** • Parallel side scissors/ 4 sets of 10 **(pg 56)** • Table crunches/ 4 sets of 10 **(pg 53)**
Day3 Slow jog 1.5 miles	**Legs and Abbs** 1. Parallel close squats/ 3 sets of 10 **(pg 49)** 2. Sumo squats/ 3 sets of 10 **(pg 48)** 3. Dumbbell lunges/ 3 sets of 10 **(pg 74)** 4. Straight leg dumbbell deadlifts/ 3 sets of 10 **(pg 77)** 5. Sumo dumbbell squats/ 3 sets of 10 **(pg 76)** (Abbs) -- • Vertical scissors / 4 sets of 10 **(pg 55)** • Single leg bridge lifts/ 4 sets of 10 (each side) **(pg 54)** • Parallel side scissors/ 4 sets of 10 **(pg 56)** • Table crunches/ 4 sets of 10 **(pg 53)**

Week 2

Cardio	Training routine
Day4 Slow jog 1.5 miles	**Arms and Abbs** 1. Single side wall pulls / 3 sets of 10 (each side) **(pg 42)** 2. Turned out dumbbell curls/ 3 sets of 10 **(pg 80)** 3. Close pushups/ 3 sets of 10 (or) hold the close pushup position 3 times. Once the burn starts, count down from 10 then stop. **(pg 47)** 4. Dumbbell curls/ 3 sets of 10 **(pg 79)** 5. Dumbbell kickbacks/ 3 sets of 10 **(pg 81)** (Abbs) -- • Vertical scissors / 4 sets of 10 **(pg 55)** • Single leg bridge lifts/ 4 sets of 10 (each side) **(pg 54)** • Parallel side scissors/ 4 sets of 10 **(pg 56)** • Table crunches/ 4 sets of 10 **(pg 53)**
Day5 Slow jog 1.5 miles	**Shoulders and Abbs** 1. Shoulder holds/ 3 times. Once the burn starts, count down from 10 then stop. **(pg 41)** 2. Dumbbell lateral raises/ 3 sets of 10 **(pg 82)** 3. Rear dumbbell raises/ 3 sets of 10 **(pg 83)** 4. Flipped dumbbell shrugs/ 3 sets of 10 **(pg 85)** 5. Military dumbbell press/ 3 sets of 10 **(pg 86)** (Abbs) -- • Vertical scissors / 3 sets of 10 **(pg 55)** • Single leg bridge lifts/ 3 sets of 10 (each side) **(pg 54)** • Parallel side scissors/ 3 sets of 10 **(pg 56)** • Table crunches/ 3 sets of 10 **(pg 53)**
Day6 **Optional** 2-3 mile walk	**Abbs** • Vertical scissors / 4 sets of 10 **(pg 55)** • Single leg bridge lifts/ 4 sets of 10 (each side) **(pg 54)** • Parallel side scissors/ 4 sets of 10 **(pg 56)** • Table crunches/ 4 sets of 10 **(pg 53)** • Leg lifts/ 3 sets of 10 **(pg 52)**
Day7 **Optional** 2-3 mile walk	**Abbs** • Vertical scissors / 4 sets of 10 **(pg 55)** • Single leg bridge lifts/ 4 sets of 15 (each side) **(pg 54)** • Parallel side scissors/ 4 sets of 15 **(pg 56)** • Table crunches/ 4 sets of 15 **(pg 53)** • Leg lifts/ 3 sets of 10 **(pg 52)**

Week 3 Cardio	Training routine
Day1 Slow jog 2 miles	**Chest and Abbs** 1. Standard pushups/ 4 sets of 10 (or) hold the pushup position 4 times. Once the burn starts, count down from 10 then stop. **(pg 45)** 2. Wide pushups/ 4 sets of 10 (or) hold the pushup position 4 times as long as possible. **(pg 46)** 3. Incline dumbbell press/ 4 sets of 10 **(pg 67)** 4. Dumbbell flys/ 4 sets of 10 **(pg 65)** 5. Dumbbell turns/ 4 sets of 10 **(pg 66)** (Abbs) -- • Vertical scissors / 4 sets of 10 **(pg 55)** • Single leg bridge lifts/ 4 sets of 10 (each side) **(pg 54)** • Parallel side scissors/ 4 sets of 10 **(pg 56)** • Leg lifts/ 4 sets of 10 **(pg 52)**
Day2 Slow jog 2 miles	**Back and Abbs** 1. Wide overhand bar pulls/ 4 sets of 10 or hold the contracted position at the top 4 times. Once the burn starts, count down from 10 then stop. **(pg 43)** 2. Turning dumbbell rows/ 4 sets of 10 **(pg 69)** 3. Wide dumbbell rows/ 4 sets of 10 **(pg 71)** 4. Standing lower back extensions/ 4 sets of 10 **(pg 50)** 5. Single dumbbell rows / 4 sets of 10 (each side) **(pg 73)** (Abbs) -- • Vertical scissors / 4 sets of 10 **(pg 55)** • Single leg bridge lifts/ 4 sets of 10 (each side) **(pg 54)** • Parallel side scissors/ 4 sets of 10 **(pg 56)** • Table crunches/ 4 sets of 10 **(pg 53)**
Day3 Slow jog 2 miles	**Legs and Abbs** 1. Parallel close squats/ 4 sets of 10 **(pg 49)** 2. Sumo squats/ 4 sets of 10 **(pg 48)** 3. Dumbbell lunges/ 4 sets of 10 **(pg 74)** 4. Straight leg dumbbell deadlifts/ 4 sets of 10 **(pg 77)** 5. Sumo dumbbell squats/ 4 sets of 10 **(pg 76)** (Abbs) -- • Vertical scissors / 4 sets of 10 **(pg 55)** • Single leg bridge lifts/ 4 sets of 10 (each side) **(pg 54)** • Parallel side scissors/ 4 sets of 10 **(pg 56)** • Table crunches/ 4 sets of 10 **(pg 53)** • Leg lifts/ 4 sets of 10 **(pg 52)**

Week 3 Cardio	Training routine
Day4 Slow jog 2 miles	**Arms and Abbs** 1. Single side wall pulls / 3 sets of 10 (each side) **(pg 42)** 2. Turned out dumbbell curls/ 4 sets of 10 **(pg 80)** 3. Close pushups/ 4 sets of 10 (or) hold the close pushup position 4 times. Once the burn starts, count down from 10 then stop. **(pg 47)** 4. Dumbbell curls/ 4 sets of 10 **(pg 79)** 5. Dumbbell kickbacks/ 4 sets of 10 **(pg 81)** (Abbs) --- • Vertical scissors / 4 sets of 10 **(pg 55)** • Single leg bridge lifts/ 4 sets of 10 (each side) **(pg 54)** • Parallel side scissors/ 4 sets of 10 **(pg 56)** • Table crunches/ 4 sets of 10 **(pg 53)** • Leg lifts/ 4 sets of 10 **(pg 52)**
Day5 Slow jog 2 miles	**Shoulders and Abbs** 1. Shoulder holds/ 4 times. Once the burn starts, count down from 10 then stop. **(pg 41)** 2. Dumbbell lateral raises/ 4 sets of 10 **(pg 82)** 3. Rear dumbbell raises/ 4 sets of 10 **(pg 83)** 4. Flipped dumbbell shrugs/ 4 sets of 10 **(pg 85)** 5. Military dumbbell press/ 4 sets of 10 **(pg 86)** (Abbs) --- • Vertical scissors / 4 sets of 10 **(pg 55)** • Single leg bridge lifts/ 4 sets of 10 (each side) **(pg 54)** • Parallel side scissors/ 4 sets of 10 **(pg 56)** • Table crunches/ 4 sets of 10 **(pg 53)** • Leg lifts/ 4 sets of 10 **(pg 52)**
Day6 **Optional** 2-3 mile walk	**Abbs** • Vertical scissors / 4 sets of 15 **(pg 55)** • Single leg bridge lifts/ 4 sets of 10 (each side) **(pg 54)** • Parallel side scissors/ 4 sets of 10 **(pg 56)** • Table crunches/ 4 sets of 10 **(pg 53)** • Leg lifts/ 3 sets of 10 **(pg 52)**
Day7 **Optional** 2-3 mile walk	**Abbs** • Vertical scissors / 4 sets of 15 **(pg 55)** • Single leg bridge lifts/ 4 sets of 15 (each side) **(pg 54)** • Parallel side scissors/ 4 sets of 15 **(pg 56)** • Table crunches/ 4 sets of 10 **(pg 53)** • Leg lifts/ 4 sets of 10 **(pg 52)**

Week 4 Cardio	Training routine
Day1 Slow jog 3 miles	• Vertical scissors / 3 sets of 10 **(pg 55)** • Single leg bridge lifts/ 3 sets of 10 (each side) **(pg 54)** • Parallel side scissors/ 3 sets of 10 **(pg 56)** • Leg lifts/ 3 sets of 10 **(pg 52)** • Table crunches/ 3 sets of 10 **(pg 53)** • Plank holds/ 3 sets/ hold the plank position 3 times. Once the burn starts, count down from 10 then stop. **(pg 57)** • Extended arm to leg lifts/ 3 sets of 10 **(pg 51)** • Dumbbell chest crunches / 3 sets of 10 **(pg 88)**
Day2 Slow jog 3 miles	• Vertical scissors / 3 sets of 10 **(pg 55)** • Single leg bridge lifts/ 3 sets of 10 (each side) **(pg 54)** • Parallel side scissors/ 3 sets of 10 **(pg 56)** • Leg lifts/ 3 sets of 10 **(pg 52)** • Table crunches/ 3 sets of 10 **(pg 53)** • Plank holds/ 3 sets/ hold the plank position 3 times. Once the burn starts, count down from 10 then stop. **(pg 57)** • Extended arm to leg lifts/ 3 sets of 10 **(pg 51)** • Dumbbell chest crunches / 3 sets of 10 **(pg 88)**
Day3 Slow jog 3 miles	• Vertical scissors / 3 sets of 10 **(pg 55)** • Single leg bridge lifts/ 3 sets of 10 (each side) **(pg 54)** • Parallel side scissors/ 3 sets of 10 **(pg 56)** • Leg lifts/ 3 sets of 10 **(pg 52)** • Table crunches/ 3 sets of 10 **(pg 53)** • Plank holds/ 3 sets / hold the plank position 3 times. Once the burn starts, count down from 10 then stop. **(pg 57)** • Extended arm to leg lifts/ 3 sets of 10 **(pg 51)** • Dumbbell chest crunches / 3 sets of 10 **(pg 88)**

Week 4 Cardio	Training routine
Day4 Slow jog 3 miles	 • Vertical scissors / 3 sets of 10 **(pg 55)** • Single leg bridge lifts/ 3 sets of 10 (each side) **(pg 54)** • Parallel side scissors/ 3 sets of 10 **(pg 56)** • Leg lifts/ 3 sets of 10 **(pg 52)** • Table crunches/ 3 sets of 10 **(pg 53)** • Plank holds/ 3 sets / hold the plank position 3 times. Once the burn starts, count down from 10 then stop. **(pg 57)** • Extended arm to leg lifts/ 3 sets of 10 **(pg 51)** • Dumbbell chest crunches / 3 sets of 10 **(pg 88)**
Day5 Slow jog 3 miles	 • Vertical scissors / 3 sets of 10 **(pg 55)** • Single leg bridge lifts/ 3 sets of 10 (each side) **(pg 54)** • Parallel side scissors/ 3 sets of 10 **(pg 56)** • Leg lifts/ 3 sets of 10 **(pg 52)** • Table crunches/ 3 sets of 10 **(pg 53)** • Plank holds/ 3 sets/ hold the plank position 3 times. Once the burn starts, count down from 10 then stop. **(pg 57)** • Extended arm to leg lifts/ 3 sets of 10 **(pg 51)** • Dumbbell chest crunches / 3 sets of 10 **(pg 88)**
Day6 **Optional** 2-4 mile walk	**Abbs** • Choose any 4 abdominal exercises from the book. Perform 4 sets of 10 repetitions per exercise. Be sure to switch sides for exercises that only hit one side of the abdominals at a time.
Day7 **Optional** 2-4 mile walk	**Abbs** • Choose any 4 abdominal exercises from the book. Perform 4 sets of 10 repetitions per exercise. Be sure to switch sides for exercises that only hit one side of the abdominals at a time.

Week 5 Cardio	Training routine
Day1 Slow jog 3 miles	**Chest and Abbs** 1. Standard pushups/ 4 sets of 12 (or) hold the pushup position 4 times. Once the burn starts, count down from 10 then stop. **(pg 45)** 2. Wide pushups/ 4 sets of 12 (or) dumbbell press/ 4 sets of 15 **(pg 46)** 3. Dumbbell flys/ 4 sets of 15 **(pg 65)** 4. Dumbbell turns/ 4 sets of 15 **(pg 66)** (Abbs) --- • Vertical scissors / 3 sets of 20 **(pg 55)** • Table crunches / 3 sets of 20 **(pg 53)** • Parallel side scissors/ 3 sets of 20 **(pg 56)**
Day2 Slow jog 3 miles	**Back and Abbs** 1. Underhand bar pulls/ 4 sets of 12 or hold the contracted position at the top 4 times. Once the burn starts, count down from 10 then stop. **(pg 44)** 2. Turning dumbbell rows/ 4 sets of 12 **(pg 69)** 3. Underhand dumbbell rows/ 4 sets of 12 **(pg 70)** 4. Standing lower back extensions/ 3 sets of 10 **(pg 50)** 5. Single dumbbell rows / 3 sets of 12 (each side) **(pg 73)** (Abbs) --- • Vertical scissors / 3 sets of 20 **(pg 55)** • Leg lifts/ 3 sets of 20 **(pg 52)** • Parallel side scissors/ 3 sets of 20 **(pg 56)** • Table crunches/ 3 sets of 20 **(pg 53)**
Day3 Slow jog 3 miles	**Legs and Abbs** 1. Parallel close squats/ 3 sets of 15 **(pg 49)** 2. Sumo squats/ 3 sets of 15 **(pg 48)** 3. Dumbbell lunges/ 3 sets of 15 **(pg 74)** 4. Straight leg dumbbell deadlifts/ 3 sets of 15 **(pg 77)** 5. Sumo dumbbell squats/ 3 sets of 15 **(pg 76)** (Abbs) --- • Vertical scissors / 3 sets of 20 **(pg 55)** • Leg lifts / 3 sets of 20 **(pg 52)** • Parallel side scissors/ 3 sets of 20 **(pg 56)** • Table crunches/ 3 sets of 20 **(pg 53)**

Week 5

Cardio	Training routine
Day4 Slow jog 3 miles	**Arms and Abbs** 1. Single side wall pulls / 3 sets of 15 each side **(pg 42)** 2. Dumbbell hammer curls/ 3 sets of 15 **(pg 78)** 3. Close pushups/ 4 sets of 10 (or) hold the pushup position 4 times. Once the burn starts, count down from 10 then stop. 4. Dumbbell curls/ 3 sets of 15 **(pg 79)** 5. Dumbbell kickbacks/ 3 sets of 12 **(pg 81)** (Abbs) -- • Vertical scissors / 3 sets of 20 **(pg 55)** • Leg lifts / 3 sets of 20 **(pg 52)** • Parallel side scissors/ 3 sets of 20 **(pg 56)** • Table crunches/ 3 sets of 20 **(pg 53)**
Day5 Slow jog 3 miles	**Shoulders and Abbs** 1. Shoulder holds/ 3 times. Once the burn starts, count down from 10 then stop. **(pg 41)** 2. Dumbbell lateral raises/ 4 sets of 12 **(pg 82)** 3. Rear dumbbell raises/ 4 sets of 12 **(pg 83)** 4. Front dumbbell raises/ 4 sets of 12 **(pg 84)** 5. Military dumbbell press/ 4 sets of 12 **(pg 86)** (Abbs) -- • Table crunches/ 10 sets of 10 **(pg 53)** or • Extended arm to leg lifts/ 8 sets of 10 **(pg 51)**
Day6 **Optional** 2-5 mile walk	**Abbs** • Vertical scissors / 5 sets of 10 **(pg 55)** • Single leg bridge lifts/ 5 sets of 10 (each side) **(pg 54)** • Parallel side scissors/ 5 sets of 10 **(pg 56)** • Table crunches/ 5 sets of 10 **(pg 53)**
Day7 **Optional** 2-5 mile walk	**Abbs** • Vertical scissors / 5 sets of 10 **(pg 55)** • Single leg bridge lifts/ 5 sets of 10 (each side) **(pg 54)** • Parallel side scissors/ 5 sets of 10 **(pg 56)** • Table crunches/ 5 sets of 10 **(pg 53)**

Week 6

Cardio	Training routine
Day1 Slow jog 3 miles	**Chest and Abbs** 1. Standard pushups/ 4 sets of 12 (or) hold the pushup position 4 times. Once the burn starts, count down from 10 then stop. **(pg 45)** 2. Wide pushups/ 4 sets of 12 (or) dumbbell press/ 4 sets of 15 **(pg 46) / (pg 64)** 3. Dumbbell flys/ 4 sets of 10 **(pg 65)** 4. Dumbbell turns/ 4 sets of 10 **(pg 66)** 5. Incline dumbbell flys/ 4 sets of 10 **(pg 68)** 6. Incline dumbbell press / 4 sets of 10 **(pg 67)** (Abbs) -- • Extended arm to leg lifts / 3 sets of 15 **(pg 51)** • Table crunches / 3 sets of 15 **(pg 53)** • Parallel side scissors/ 3 sets of 20 **(pg 56)**
Day2 Slow jog 3 miles	**Back and Abbs** 1. Underhand bar pulls/ 4 sets of 10 or hold the contracted position at the top 4 times. Once the burn starts, count down from 10 then stop. **(pg 44)** 2. Turning dumbbell rows/ 4 sets of 12 **(pg 69)** 3. Underhand dumbbell rows/ 4 sets of 12 **(pg 70)** 4. Standing lower back extensions/ 3 sets of 10 **(pg 50)** 5. Single dumbbell rows / 3 sets of 12 (each side) **(pg 73)** 6. Wide over hand bar pulls/ 3 sets of 10 **(pg 43)** (Abbs) -- • Leg lifts/ 4 sets of 15 **(pg 52)** • Parallel side scissors/ 3 sets of 20 **(pg 56)** • Table crunches/ 4 sets of 15 **(pg 53)**
Day3 Slow jog 3 miles	**Legs and Abbs** 1. Parallel close squats/ 3 sets of 15 **(pg 49)** 2. Sumo squats/ 3 sets of 15 **(pg 48)** 3. Dumbbell lunges/ 3 sets of 15 **(pg 74)** 4. Straight leg dumbbell deadlifts/ 3 sets of 15 **(pg 77)** 5. Sumo dumbbell squats/ 3 sets of 15 **(pg 76)** 6. Parallel dumbbell squats/ 3 sets of 10 **(pg 75)** (Abbs) -- • Vertical scissors / 3 sets of 20 **(pg 55)** • Leg lifts / 3 sets of 20 (each side) **(pg 52)** • Parallel side scissors/ 3 sets of 20 **(pg 56)** • Table crunches/ 3 sets of 20 **(pg 53)**

Week 6

Cardio	Training routine

Day4
 	
Slow jog
3 miles
	Arms and Abbs
	1. Dumbbell hammer curls/ 3 sets of 15 **(pg 78)**
	2. Close pushups/ 4 sets of 15 (or) hold the close pushup position 4 times. Once the burn starts, count down from 10 then stop. **(pg 47)**
	3. Dumbbell curls/ 3 sets of 15 **(pg 79)**
	4. Dumbbell kickbacks/ 3 sets of 12 **(pg 81)**
	5. Turned out dumbbell curls/ 3 sets of 15 **(pg 80)**
	(Abbs) --
	    • Leg lifts / 4 sets of 20 **(pg 52)**
	    • Table crunches/ 4 sets of 20 **(pg 53)**
	    • Extended arm to leg lifts / 3 sets of 15 **(pg 51)**

Day5
 	
Slow jog
3 miles
	Shoulders and Abbs
	6. Shoulder holds/ 4 times. Once the burn starts, count down from 15 then stop. **(pg 41)**
	7. Dumbbell lateral raises/ 4 sets of 15 **(pg 82)**
	8. Rear dumbbell raises/ 4 sets of 15 **(pg 83)**
	9. Front dumbbell raises/ 4 sets of 15 **(pg 84)**
	10. Military dumbbell press/ 4 sets of 15 **(pg 86)**
	(Abbs) --
	    • Table crunches/ 10 sets of 15 **(pg 53)**
	                or
	    • Extended arm to leg lifts/ 8 sets of 12 **(pg 51)**

Day6
Optional
 	
2-5 mile walk
	Abbs
	    • Vertical scissors / 5 sets of 10 **(pg 55)**
	    • Single leg bridge lifts/ 5 sets of 10 (each side) **(pg 54)**
	    • Parallel side scissors/ 5 sets of 10 **(pg 56)**
	    • Table crunches/ 5 sets of 10 **(pg 53)**

Day7
Optional
2-5 mile walk
	Abbs
	    • Vertical scissors / 5 sets of 10 **(pg 55)**
	    • Single leg bridge lifts/ 5 sets of 10 (each side) **(pg 54)**
	    • Parallel side scissors/ 5 sets of 10 **(pg 56)**
	    • Table crunches/ 5 sets of 10 **(pg 53)**

Week 7 Cardio	Training routine

<u>Day1</u>
 	
Slow jog
3 miles
	• Standing side crunches/ 3 sets of 10 (each side) **(pg 58)**
	• Vertical scissors / 3 sets of 10 **(pg 55)**
	• Single leg bridge lifts/ 3 sets of 10 (each side) **(pg 54)**
	• Parallel side scissors/ 3 sets of 10 **(pg 56)**
	• Leg lifts/ 3 sets of 10 **(pg 52)**
	• Table crunches/ 3 sets of 10 **(pg 53)**
	• Plank holds/ 3 sets/ hold the plank position 3 times.
	   Once the burn starts, count down from 10 then stop.
	   (pg 57)
	• Extended arm to leg lifts/ 3 sets of 10 **(pg 51)**
	• Dumbbell chest crunches / 3 sets of 10 **(pg 88)**

<u>Day2</u>
 	
Slow jog
3 miles
	• Standing side crunches/ 3 sets of 10 (each side) **(pg 58)**
	• Vertical scissors / 3 sets of 10 **(pg 55)**
	• Single leg bridge lifts/ 3 sets of 10 (each side) **(pg 54)**
	• Parallel side scissors/ 3 sets of 10 **(pg 56)**
	• Leg lifts/ 3 sets of 10 **(pg 52)**
	• Table crunches/ 3 sets of 10 **(pg 53)**
	• Plank holds/ 3 sets/ hold the plank position 3 times.
	   Once the burn starts, count down from 10 then stop.
	   (pg 57)
	• Extended arm to leg lifts/ 3 sets of 10 **(pg 51)**
	• Dumbbell chest crunches / 3 sets of 10 **(pg 88)**

<u>Day3</u>
 	
Slow jog
3 miles
	• Standing side crunches/ 3 sets of 10 (each side) **(pg 58)**
	• Vertical scissors / 3 sets of 10 **(pg 55)**
	• Single leg bridge lifts/ 3 sets of 10 (each side) **(pg 54)**
	• Parallel side scissors/ 3 sets of 10 **(pg 56)**
	• Leg lifts/ 3 sets of 10 **(pg 52)**
	• Table crunches/ 3 sets of 10 **(pg 53)**
	• Plank holds/ 3 sets / hold the plank position 3 times.
	   Once the burn starts, count down from 10 then stop.
	   (pg 57)
	• Extended arm to leg lifts/ 3 sets of 10 **(pg 51)**
	• Dumbbell chest crunches / 3 sets of 10 **(pg 88)**

Week 7 Cardio	Training routine
Day4 Slow jog 3 miles	• Standing side crunches/ 3 sets of 10 (each side) **(pg 58)** • Vertical scissors / 3 sets of 10 **(pg 55)** • Single leg bridge lifts/ 3 sets of 10 (each side) **(pg 54)** • Parallel side scissors/ 3 sets of 10 **(pg 56)** • Leg lifts/ 3 sets of 10 **(pg 52)** • Table crunches/ 3 sets of 10 **(pg 53)** • Plank holds/ 3 sets / hold the plank position 3 times. Once the burn starts, count down from 10 then stop. **(pg 57)** • Extended arm to leg lifts/ 3 sets of 10 **(pg 51)** • Dumbbell chest crunches / 3 sets of 10 **(pg 88)**
Day5 Slow jog 3 miles	• Standing side crunches/ 3 sets of 10 (each side) **(pg 58)** • Vertical scissors / 3 sets of 10 **(pg 55)** • Single leg bridge lifts/ 3 sets of 10 (each side) **(pg 54)** • Parallel side scissors/ 3 sets of 10 **(pg 56)** • Leg lifts/ 3 sets of 10 **(pg 52)** • Table crunches/ 3 sets of 10 **(pg 53)** • Plank holds/ 3 sets/ hold the plank position 3 times. Once the burn starts, count down from 10 then stop. **(pg 57)** • Extended arm to leg lifts/ 3 sets of 10 **(pg 51)** • Dumbbell chest crunches / 3 sets of 10 **(pg 88)**
Day6 Optional 2-4 mile walk	**Abbs** • Vertical scissors / 4 sets of 15 **(pg 55)** • Single leg bridge lifts/ 4 sets of 10 (each side) **(pg 54)** • Parallel side scissors/ 4 sets of 10 **(pg 56)** • Table crunches/ 4 sets of 10 **(pg 53)** • Leg lifts/ 4 sets of 10 **(pg 52)**
Day7 Optional 2-4 mile walk	**Abbs** • Vertical scissors / 4 sets of 15 **(pg 55)** • Single leg bridge lifts/ 4 sets of 15 (each side) **(pg 54)** • Parallel side scissors/ 4 sets of 15 **(pg 56)** • Table crunches/ 4 sets of 10 **(pg 53)** • Leg lifts/ 4 sets of 10 **(pg 52)**

Week 8

Cardio	Training routine
Day1 Slow jog 3 miles	**Chest and Abbs** 1. Standard pushups/ 4 sets of 15 (or) hold the pushup position 4 times. Once the burn starts, count down from 12 then stop. **(pg 45)** 2. Wide pushups/ 3 sets of 10 (or) hold the wide pushup position 3 times as long as possible. **(pg 46)** 3. Dumbbell press/ 5 sets of 20 **(pg 64)** 4. Dumbbell flys/ 5 sets of 20 **(pg 65)** 5. Dumbbell turns/ 5 sets of 20 **(pg 66)** (Abbs) --- • Vertical scissors / 3 sets of 25 **(pg 55)** • Parallel side scissors/ 3 sets of 25 **(pg 56)** • Leg lifts/ 3 sets of 25 **(pg 52)**
Day2 Slow jog 3 miles	**Back and Abbs** 1. Underhand bar pulls/ 4 sets of 10 or hold the contracted position at the top 4 times. Once the burn starts, count down from 10 then stop. **(pg 44)** 2. Turning dumbbell rows/ 5 sets of 20 **(pg 69)** 3. Underhand dumbbell rows/ 5 sets of 20 **(pg 70)** 4. Standing lower back extensions/ 4 sets of 10 **(pg 50)** 5. Single dumbbell rows / 3 sets of 20 (each side) **(pg 73)** (Abbs) --- • Vertical scissors / 3 sets of 20 **(pg 55)** • Single leg bridge lifts/ 3 sets of 20 (each side) **(pg 54)** • Parallel side scissors/ 3 sets of 20 **(pg 56)** • Table crunches/ 3 sets of 20 **(pg 53)**
Day3 Slow jog 3 miles	**Legs and Abbs** 1. Parallel close squats/ 4 sets of 20 **(pg 49)** 2. Sumo squats/ 4 sets of 20 **(pg 48)** 3. Dumbbell lunges/ 3 sets of 15 **(pg 74)** 4. Straight leg dumbbell deadlifts/ 3 sets of 15 **(pg 77)** 5. Sumo dumbbell squats/ 3 sets of 20 **(pg 76)** (Abbs) --- • Vertical scissors / 3 sets of 10 **(pg 55)** • Single leg bridge lifts/ 3 sets of 10 (each side) **(pg 54)** • Parallel side scissors/ 3 sets of 10 **(pg 56)** • Table crunches/ 3 sets of 10 **(pg 53)** • Abdominal exhales/ 3 sets of 10 **(pg 60)**

Week 8 Cardio	Training routine
Day4 Slow jog 3 miles	**Arms and Abbs** 1. Single side wall pulls / 3 sets of 20 (each side) **(pg 42)** 2. Dumbbell hammer curls/ 3 sets of 20 **(pg 78)** 3. Close pushups/ 3 sets of 20 (or) hold the close pushup position 3 times. Once the burn starts, count down from 15 then stop. **(pg 47)** 4. Dumbbell curls/ 3 sets of 20 **(pg 79)** 5. Dumbbell kickbacks/ 3 sets of 20 **(pg 81)** (Abbs) -- • Extended arm to leg lifts/ 5 sets of 15 **(pg 51)** • Single leg bridge lifts/ 3 sets of 10 (each side) **(pg 54)** • Table crunches/ 5 sets of 10 **(pg 53)**
Day5 Slow jog 3 miles	**Shoulders and Abbs** 1. Shoulder holds/ 3 times. Once the burn starts, count down from 20 then stop. **(pg 41)** 2. Dumbbell lateral raises/ 4 sets of 20 **(pg 82)** 3. Rear dumbbell raises/ 4 sets of 20 **(pg 83)** 4. Front dumbbell raises/ 4 sets of 15 **(pg 84)** 5. Military dumbbell press/ 4 sets of 15 **(pg 86)** (Abbs) -- • Muay Thai knee/ 3 sets of 10 (each side) **(pg 59)** • Vertical scissors / 3 sets of 10 **(pg 55)** • Single leg bridge lifts/ 3 sets of 10 (each side) **(pg 54)** • Parallel side scissors/ 3 sets of 10 **(pg 56)** • Table crunches/ 3 sets of 10 **(pg 53)**
Day6 **Optional** 2-3 mile walk	**Abbs** • Choose any 4 abdominal exercises from the book. Perform 4 sets of 10 repetitions per exercise. Be sure to switch sides for exercises that only hit one side of the abdominals at a time.
Day7 **Optional** 2-3 mile walk	**Abbs** • Choose any 4 abdominal exercises from the book. Perform 4 sets of 10 repetitions per exercise. Be sure to switch sides for exercises that only hit one side of the abdominals at a time.

Week 9

Cardio	Training routine
Day1 Slow jog 3-4 miles	**Chest and Abbs** 1. Standard pushups/ 5 sets of 10 (or) hold the pushup position 3 times. Once the burn starts, count down from 20 then stop. **(pg 45)** 2. Wide pushups/ 5 sets of 10 (or) hold the wide pushup position 5 times as long as possible. **(pg 46)** 3. Incline dumbbell press/ 5 sets of 25 **(pg 67)** 4. Incline dumbbell flys/ 5 sets of 25 **(pg 68)** 5. Dumbbell turns/ 5 sets of 25 **(pg 66)** (Abbs) -- • Choose any 4 abdominal exercises from the book. Perform 4 sets of 15 repetitions per exercise. Be sure to switch sides for exercises that only hit one side of the abdominals at a time.
Day2 Slow jog 3-4 miles	**Back and Abbs** 1. Wide overhand bar pulls/ 5 sets of 15 (or) hold the contracted position at the top 4 times. Once the burn starts, count down from 15 then stop. **(pg 43)** 2. Turning dumbbell rows/ 4 sets of 25 **(pg 69)** 3. Wide dumbbell rows/ 4 sets of 25 **(pg 71)** 4. Standing lower back extensions/ 4 sets of 10 **(pg 50)** 5. Single dumbbell rows / 3 sets of 20 (each side) **(pg 73)** (Abbs) -- • Vertical scissors / 4 sets of 25 **(pg 55)** • Single leg bridge lifts/ 4 sets of 20 (each side) **(pg 54)** • Parallel side scissors/ 4 sets of 25 **(pg 56)** • Table crunches/ 4 sets of 20 **(pg 53)**
Day3 Slow jog 3-4 miles	**Legs and Abbs** 1. Parallel close squats/ 4 sets of 25 **(pg 49)** 2. Sumo squats/ 4 sets of 25 **(pg 48)** 3. Dumbbell lunges/ 3 sets of 15 **(pg 74)** 4. Straight leg dumbbell deadlifts/ 3 sets of 15 **(pg 77)** 5. Sumo dumbbell squats/ 2 sets of 20 **(pg 76)** 6. Calf raises/ 4 sets of 10 **(pg 61)** (Abbs) -- • Vertical scissors / 4 sets of 25 **(pg 55)** • Single leg bridge lifts/ 4 sets of 20 (each side) **(pg 54)** • Parallel side scissors/ 4 sets of 25 **(pg 56)** • Table crunches/ 4 sets of 25 **(pg 53)**

Week 9 Cardio	Training routine
Day4 Slow jog 3-4 miles	**Arms and Abbs** 1. Turned out dumbbell curls/ 4 sets of 20 **(pg 80)** 2. Close pushups/ 4 sets of 15 (or) hold the close pushup position 4 times. Once the burn starts, count down from 15 then stop. **(pg 47)** 3. Dumbbell curls/ 4 sets of 25 **(pg 79)** 4. Dumbbell kickbacks/ 6 sets of 12 **(pg 81)** (Abbs) --- • Table crunches/ 5 sets of 20 **(pg 53)** • Leg lifts/ 5 sets of 20 **(pg 52)**
Day5 Slow jog 3-4 miles	**Shoulders and Abbs** 1. Shoulder holds/ 4 times. Once the burn starts, count down from 15 then stop. **(pg 41)** 2. Dumbbell lateral raises/ 4 sets of 20 **(pg 82)** 3. Rear dumbbell raises/ 3 sets of 15 **(pg 83)** 4. Flipped dumbbell shrugs/ 3 sets of 20 **(pg 85)** 5. Military dumbbell press/ 4 sets of 15 **(pg 86)** (Abbs) --- • Table crunches/ 5 sets of 20 **(pg 53)** • Muay Thai knee/ 5 sets of 10 (each side) **(pg 59)**
Day6 **Optional** 2-3 mile walk	**Abbs** • Choose any 4 abdominal exercises from the book. Perform 4 sets of 15 repetitions per exercise. Be sure to switch sides for exercises that only hit one side of the abdominals at a time.
Day7 **Optional** 2-3 mile walk	**Abbs** • Vertical scissors / 4 sets of 10 **(pg 55)** • Single leg bridge lifts/ 4 sets of 15 (each side) **(pg 54)** • Parallel side scissors/ 4 sets of 15 **(pg 56)** • Table crunches/ 4 sets of 15 **(pg 53)** • Leg lifts/ 3 sets of 10 **(pg 52)**

Week 10 Cardio	Training routine
Day1 Slow jog 4 miles	<ul><li>Vertical scissors / 3 sets of 10 **(pg 55)**</li><li>Muay Thai knee/ 3 sets of 10 (each side) **(pg 59)**</li><li>Dumbbell single leg mini crunches 3 sets of 10 (each side) **(pg 89)**</li><li>Leg lifts/ 3 sets of 10 **(pg 52)**</li><li>Table crunches/ 3 sets of 10 **(pg 53)**</li><li>Plank holds/ 3 sets/ hold the plank position 3 times. Once the burn starts, count down from 20 then stop. **(pg 57)**</li><li>Extended arm to leg lifts/ 3 sets of 10 **(pg 51)**</li><li>Dumbbell chest crunches / 3 sets of 10 **(pg 88)**</li></ul>
Day2 Slow jog 4 miles	<ul><li>Vertical scissors / 3 sets of 10 **(pg 55)**</li><li>Muay Thai knee/ 3 sets of 10 (each side) **(pg 59)**</li><li>Dumbbell single leg mini crunches 3 sets of 10 (each side) **(pg 89)**</li><li>Leg lifts/ 3 sets of 10 **(pg 52)**</li><li>Table crunches/ 3 sets of 10 **(pg 53)**</li><li>Abdominal exhales / 3 sets of 10 **(pg 60)**</li><li>Extended arm to leg lifts/ 3 sets of 10 **(pg 51)**</li><li>Dumbbell chest crunches / 3 sets of 10 **(pg 88)**</li><li>Dumbbell table crunches/ 3 sets of 10 **(pg 87)**</li></ul>
Day3 Slow jog 4 miles	<ul><li>Vertical scissors / 3 sets of 10 **(pg 55)**</li><li>Muay Thai knee/ 3 sets of 10 (each side) **(pg 59)**</li><li>Dumbbell single leg mini crunches 3 sets of 10 (each side) **(pg 89)**</li><li>Leg lifts/ 3 sets of 10 **(pg 52)**</li><li>Table crunches/ 3 sets of 10 **(pg 53)**</li><li>Plank holds/ 3 sets/ hold the plank position 3 times. Once the burn starts, count down from 20 then stop. **(pg 57)**</li><li>Extended arm to leg lifts/ 3 sets of 10 **(pg 51)**</li><li>Dumbbell chest crunches / 3 sets of 10 **(pg 88)**</li></ul>

Week 10
Cardio   **Training routine**

Day4 Slow jog 4 miles	• Vertical scissors / 3 sets of 10 **(pg 55)** • Muay Thai knee/ 3 sets of 10 (each side) **(pg 59)** • Dumbbell single leg mini crunches 3 sets of 10 (each side) **(pg 89)** • Leg lifts/ 3 sets of 10 **(pg 52)** • Table crunches/ 3 sets of 10 **(pg 53)** • Abdominal exhales / 3 sets of 10 **(pg 60)** • Extended arm to leg lifts/ 3 sets of 10 **(pg 51)** • Dumbbell chest crunches / 3 sets of 10 **(pg 88)** • Dumbbell table crunches/ 3 sets of 10 **(pg 87)**
Day5 Slow jog 4 miles	• Vertical scissors / 3 sets of 10 **(pg 55)** • Single leg bridge lifts/ 3 sets of 10 (each side) **(pg 54)** • Parallel side scissors/ 3 sets of 10 **(pg 56)** • Leg lifts/ 3 sets of 10 **(pg 52)** • Table crunches/ 3 sets of 10 **(pg 53)** • Plank holds/ 3 sets/ hold the plank position 3 times. Once the burn starts, count down from 10 then stop. **(pg 57)** • Extended arm to leg lifts/ 3 sets of 10 **(pg 51)** • Dumbbell chest crunches / 3 sets of 10 **(pg 88)**
Day6 **Optional** 2-4 mile walk	**Abbs** • Choose any 5 abdominal exercises from the book. Perform 4 sets of 10 repetitions per exercise. Be sure to switch sides for exercises that only hit one side of the abdominals at a time.
Day7 **Optional** 2-4 mile walk	**Abbs** • Choose any 5 abdominal exercises from the book. Perform 4 sets of 10 repetitions per exercise. Be sure to switch sides for exercises that only hit one side of the abdominals at a time.

Week 11

Cardio	Training routine
Day1 Slow jog 4 miles	**Chest and Abbs** 1. Dumbbell press/ 4 sets of 25 **(pg 64)** 2. Dumbbell flys/ 4 sets of 25 **(pg 65)** 3. Dumbbell turns/ 4 sets of 25 **(pg 66)** 4. Incline dumbbell press/ 2 sets of 25 **(pg 67)** 5. Incline dumbbell flys/ 2 sets of 25 **(pg 68)** (Abbs) --- • Leg lifts / 5 sets of 20 **(pg 52)** • Plank Holds/ 4 sets/ hold the plank position 4 times. Once the burn starts, count down from 20 then stop. **(pg 57)** • Table crunches/ 5 sets of 20 **(pg 53)**
Day2 Slow jog 4 miles	**Back and Abbs** 1. Underhand bar pulls/ 3 sets of 20 **(pg 44)** 2. Turning dumbbell rows/ 3 sets of 20 **(pg 69)** 3. Underhand dumbbell rows/ 3 sets of 20 **(pg 44)** 4. Wide overhand bar pulls / 3 sets of 20 **(pg 43)** 5. Standing lower back extensions/ 3 sets of 15 **(pg 50)** 6. Single dumbbell rows / 3 sets of 20 (each side) **(pg 73)** (Abbs) --- • Vertical scissors / 3 sets of 25 **(pg 55)** • Parallel side scissors/ 3 sets of 25 **(pg 56)** • Table crunches/ 5 scts of 20 **(pg 53)** • Extended arm to leg lifts/ 3 sets of 15 **(pg 51)**
Day3 Slow jog 4 miles	**Legs and Abbs** 1. Parallel close squats/ 3 sets of 25 **(pg 49)** 2. Sumo squats/ 3 sets of 20 **(pg 48)** 3. Dumbbell lunges/ 3 sets of 15 **(pg 74)** 4. Straight leg dumbbell deadlifts/ 4 sets of 12 **(pg 77)** 5. Sumo dumbbell squats/ 4 sets of 12 **(pg 76)** 6. Calf raises/ 4 sets of 20 **(pg 61)** (Abbs) --- • Leg lifts / 5 sets of 20 **(pg 52)** • Plank holds/ 4 sets/ hold the plank position 4 times. Once the burn starts, count down from 20 then stop. **(pg 57)** • Table crunches/ 5 sets of 20 **(pg 53)** • Muay Thai knee/ 3 sets of 15 (each side) **(pg 59)**

Week 11 Cardio	Training routine
Day4 Slow jog 4 miles	**Arms and Abbs** 1. Dumbbell hammer curls/ 5 sets of 20 **(pg 78)** 2. Close pushups/ 5 sets of 10 (or) hold the close pushup position 5 times. Once the burn starts, count down from 15 then stop. **(pg 47)** 3. Dumbbell curls/ 5 sets of 20 **(pg 79)** 4. Dumbbell kickbacks/ 5 sets of 10 **(pg 81)** (Abbs) --- • Vertical scissors / 3 sets of 10 **(pg 55)** • Single leg bridge lifts/ 3 sets of 10 (each side) **(pg 54)** • Parallel side scissors/ 3 sets of 10 **(pg 56)** • Table crunches/ 3 sets of 10 **(pg 53)**
Day5 Slow jog 4 miles	**Shoulders and Abbs** 1. Shoulder holds/ 5 times. Once the burn starts, count down from 15 then stop. **(pg 41)** 2. Dumbbell lateral raises/ 5 sets of 20 **(pg 82)** 3. Rear dumbbell raises/ 5 sets of 15 **(pg 83)** 4. Front dumbbell raises/ 4 sets of 15 **(pg 84)** 5. Military dumbbell press/ 5 sets of 12 **(pg 86)** (Abbs) --- • Leg lifts / 5 sets of 20 **(pg 52)** • Plank holds/ 4 sets/ hold the plank position 4 times. Once the burn starts, count down from 15 then stop. **(pg 57)** • Table crunches/ 5 sets of 20 **(pg 53)** • Muay Thai knee/ 3 sets of 10 (each side) **(pg 59)**
Day6 **Optional** 3-5 mile walk	**Abbs** • Choose any 5 abdominal exercises from the book. Perform 4 sets of 12 repetitions per exercise. Be sure to switch sides for exercises that only hit one side of the abdominals at a time.
Day7 **Optional** 3-5 mile walk	**Abbs** • Choose any 5 abdominal exercises from the book. Perform 4 sets of 12 repetitions per exercise. Be sure to switch sides for exercises that only hit one side of the abdominals at a time.

Week 12 Cardio	Training routine
Day1 Slow jog 4 miles	**The Mix up** 1. Dumbbell press/ 4 sets of 20 **(pg 64)** 2. Turning dumbbell rows/ 4 sets of 20 **(pg 69)** 3. Parallel dumbbell squats/ 4 sets of 20 **(pg 75)** 4. Dumbbell hammer curls/ 4 sets of 20 **(pg 78)** 5. Dumbbell lateral raises/ 4 sets of 20 **(pg 82)** (Abbs) -- • Leg lifts / 5 sets of 20 **(pg 52)** • Plank holds/ 4 sets/ hold the plank position 4 times. Once the burn starts, count down from 20 then stop. **(pg 57)** • Table crunches/ 5 sets of 25 **(pg 53)**
Day2 Slow jog 4 miles	**The Mix up** 1. Dumbbell flys/ 4 sets of 20 **(pg 65)** 2. Underhand dumbbell rows/ 4 sets of 20 **(pg 70)** 3. Dumbbell kickbacks / 4 sets of 20 **(pg 81)** 4. Dumbbell lunges / 4 sets of 20 **(pg 74)** 5. Flipped dumbbell shrugs/ 4 sets of 20 **(pg 85)** (Abbs) -- • Vertical scissors / 3 sets of 25 **(pg 55)** • Parallel side scissors/ 3 sets of 25 **(pg 56)** • Table crunches/ 5 sets of 20 **(pg 53)** • Extended arm to leg lifts/ 4 sets of 15 **(pg 51)**
Day3 Slow jog 4 miles	**Legs and Abbs** 1. Parallel close squats/ 3 sets of 25 **(pg 49)** 2. Sumo squats/ 3 sets of 20 **(pg 48)** 3. Dumbbell lunges/ 3 sets of 15 **(pg 74)** 4. Straight leg dumbbell deadlifts/ 4 sets of 12 **(pg 77)** 5. Sumo dumbbell squats/ 4 sets of 12 **(pg 76)** 6. Calf raises/ 4 sets of 20 **(pg 61)** (Abbs) -- • Leg lifts / 5 sets of 20 **(pg 52)** • Plank holds/ 4 sets/ hold the plank position 4 times. Once the burn starts, count down from 15 then stop. **(pg 57)** • Table crunches/ 5 sets of 20 **(pg 53)** • Muay Thai knee/ 3 sets of 10 (each side) **(pg 59)**

Week 12
Cardio   **Training routine**

Day	Cardio	Training routine
Day4	Slow jog 4 miles	**Arms and Abbs** 1. Dumbbell hammer curls/ 5 sets of 20 **(pg 78)** 2. Close pushups/ 5 sets of 15 (or) hold the close pushup position 5 times. Once the burn starts, count down from 15 then stop. **(pg 47)** 3. Dumbbell curls/ 5 sets of 20 **(pg 79)** 4. Dumbbell kickbacks/ 5 sets of 10 **(pg 81)** (Abbs) --- • Vertical scissors / 3 sets of 20 **(pg 55)** • Single leg bridge lifts/ 3 sets of 20 (each side) **(pg 54)** • Parallel side scissors/ 3 sets of 20 **(pg 56)** • Table crunches/ 3 sets of 20 **(pg 53)**
Day5	Slow jog 4 miles	**Shoulders and Abbs** 1. Shoulder holds/ 5 times. Once the burn starts, count down from 15 then stop. **(pg 41)** 2. Dumbbell lateral raises/ 5 sets of 20 **(pg 82)** 3. Rear dumbbell raises/ 5 sets of 15 **(pg 83)** 4. Front dumbbell raises/ 4 sets of 15 **(pg 84)** 5. Military dumbbell press/ 5 sets of 15 **(pg 86)** (Abbs) --- • Leg lifts / 5 sets of 20 **(pg 52)** • Plank holds/ 4 sets/ hold the plank position 4 times. Once the burn starts, count down from 15 then stop. **(pg 57)** • Table crunches/ 5 sets of 20 **(pg 53)** • Muay Thai knee/ 3 sets of 10 (each side) **(pg 59)**
Day6 **Optional** 3-5 mile walk		**Abbs** • Choose any 5 abdominal exercises from the book. Perform 4 sets of 12 repetitions per exercise. Be sure to switch sides for exercises that only hit one side of the abdominals at a time.
Day7 **Optional** 3-5 mile walk		**Abbs** • Choose any 5 abdominal exercises from the book. Perform 4 sets of 12 repetitions per exercise. Be sure to switch sides for exercises that only hit one side of the abdominals at a time.

Week 13 Cardio	Training routine
<u>Day1</u> Slow jog 4 miles	• Vertical scissors / 3 sets of 10 **(pg 55)** • Muay Thai knee/ 3 sets of 10 (each side) **(pg 59)** • Dumbbell single leg mini crunches 3 sets of 10 (each side) **(pg 89)** • Leg lifts/ 3 sets of 10 **(pg 52)** • Table crunches/ 3 sets of 10 **(pg 53)** • Plank holds/ 3 sets/ hold the plank position 3 times. Once the burn starts, count down from 10 then stop. **(pg 57)** • Extended arm to leg lifts/ 3 sets of 10 **(pg 51)** • Dumbbell chest crunches / 3 sets of 10 **(pg 88)**
<u>Day2</u> Slow jog 4 miles	• Vertical scissors / 3 sets of 10 **(pg 55)** • Muay Thai knee/ 3 sets of 10 (each side) **(pg 59)** • Dumbbell single leg mini crunches 3 sets of 10 (each side) **(pg 89)** • Leg lifts/ 3 sets of 10 **(pg 52)** • Table crunches/ 3 sets of 10 **(pg 53)** • Abdominal exhales / 3 sets of 10 **(pg 60)** • Extended arm to leg lifts/ 3 sets of 10 **(pg 51)** • Dumbbell chest crunches / 3 sets of 10 **(pg 88)** • Dumbbell table crunches/ 3 sets of 10 **(pg 87)**
<u>Day3</u> Slow jog 4 miles	• Vertical scissors / 3 sets of 10 **(pg 55)** • Muay Thai knee/ 3 sets of 10 (each side) **(pg 59)** • Dumbbell single leg mini crunches 3 sets of 10 (each side) **(pg 89)** • Leg lifts/ 3 sets of 10 **(pg 52)** • Table crunches/ 3 sets of 10 **(pg 53)** • Plank holds/ 3 sets/ hold the plank position 3 times. Once the burn starts, count down from 10 then stop. **(pg 57)** • Extended arm to leg lifts/ 3 sets of 10 **(pg 51)** • Dumbbell chest crunches / 3 sets of 10 **(pg 88)**

Week 13 Cardio	Training routine
Day4 Slow jog 4 miles	• Vertical scissors / 3 sets of 10 **(pg 55)** • Muay Thai knee/ 3 sets of 10 (each side) **(pg 59)** • Dumbbell single leg mini crunches 3 sets of 10 (each side) **(pg 89)** • Leg lifts/ 3 sets of 10 **(pg 52)** • Table crunches/ 3 sets of 10 **(pg 53)** • Abdominal exhales / 3 sets of 10 **(pg 60)** • Extended arm to leg lifts/ 3 sets of 10 **(pg 51)** • Dumbbell chest crunches / 3 sets of 10 **(pg 88)** • Dumbbell table crunches/ 3 sets of 10 **(pg 87)**
Day5 Slow jog 4 miles	• Vertical scissors / 3 sets of 10 **(pg 55)** • Single leg bridge lifts/ 3 sets of 10 (each side) **(pg 54)** • Parallel side scissors/ 3 sets of 10 **(pg 56)** • Leg lifts/ 3 sets of 10 **(pg 52)** • Table crunches/ 3 sets of 10 **(pg 53)** • Plank holds/ 3 sets/ hold the plank position 3 times. Once the burn starts, count down from 10 then stop. **(pg 57)** • Extended arm to leg lifts/ 3 sets of 10 **(pg 51)** • Dumbbell chest crunches / 3 sets of 10 **(pg 88)**
Day6 **Optional** 2-4 mile walk	**Abbs** • Choose any 5 abdominal exercises from the book. Perform 4 sets of 12 repetitions per exercise. Be sure to switch sides for exercises that only hit one side of the abdominals at a time.
Day7 **Optional** 2-4 mile walk	**Abbs** • Choose any 5 abdominal exercises from the book. Perform 4 sets of 12 repetitions per exercise. Be sure to switch sides for exercises that only hit one side of the abdominals at a time.

Week 14

Cardio	Training routine

Day1
 	
Slow jog
4 miles
	The Mix up
	1. Dumbbell press/ 4 sets of 20 **(pg 64)**
	2. Turning dumbbell rows/ 4 sets of 20 **(pg 69)**
	3. Parallel dumbbell squats/ 4 sets of 20 **(pg 75)**
	4. Dumbbell hammer curls/ 4 sets of 20 **(pg 78)**
	5. Dumbbell lateral raises/ 4 sets of 20 **(pg 82)**
	(Abbs) ---
	• Leg lifts / 5 sets of 20 **(pg 52)**
	• Plank holds/ 4 sets/ hold the plank position 4 times.
	  Once the burn starts, count down from 20 then stop.
	  (pg 57)
	• Table crunches/ 5 sets of 25 **(pg 53)**

Day2 Slow jog 4 miles	**The Mix up** 1. Dumbbell flys/ 4 sets of 20 **(pg 65)** 2. Underhand dumbbell rows/ 4 sets of 20 **(pg 70)** 3. Dumbbell kickbacks / 4 sets of 20 **(pg 81)** 4. Dumbbell lunges / 4 sets of 20 **(pg 74)** 5. Flipped dumbbell shrugs/ 4 sets of 20 **(pg 85)** (Abbs) --- • Vertical scissors / 3 sets of 25 **(pg 55)** • Parallel side scissors/ 3 sets of 25 **(pg 56)** • Table crunches/ 5 sets of 20 **(pg 53)** • Extended arm to leg lifts/ 3 sets of 15 **(pg 51)**

Day3
 	
Slow jog
4 miles
	The Mix up
	1. Incline dumbbell press/ 4 sets of 20 **(pg 67)**
	2. Underhand bar pulls/ 4 sets of 20 **(pg 44)**
	3. Close pushups/ 5 sets of 10 **(pg 47)**
	4. Straight leg dumbbell deadlifts/ 4 sets of 12 **(pg 77)**
	5. Rear dumbbell lateral raises/ 4 sets of 15 **(pg 83)**
	6. Calf raises/ 4 sets of 20 **(pg 61)**
	(Abbs) ---
	• Leg lifts / 5 sets of 20 **(pg 52)**
	• Plank holds/ 4 sets/ hold the plank position 4 times.
	  Once the burn starts, count down from 20 then stop.
	  (pg 57)
	• Table crunches/ 5 sets of 20 **(pg 53)**
	• Muay Thai knee/ 3 sets of 10 (each side) **(pg 59)**

Week 14

Cardio	Training routine

Day4
 	
Slow jog
4 miles
	The Mix up
	1. Dumbbell curls/ 5 sets of 20 **(pg 79)**
	2. Close pushups/ 5 sets of 10 (or) hold the close pushup position 5 times. Once the burn starts, count down from 15 then stop. **(pg 47)**
	3. Sumo squats/ 5 sets of 25 **(pg 48)**
	4. Military dumbbell press/ 4 sets of 15 **(pg 86)**
	(Abbs) --
	  • Vertical scissors / 4 sets of 20 **(pg 55)**
	  • Single leg bridge lifts/ 4 sets of 20 (each side) **(pg 54)**
	  • Parallel side scissors/ 4 sets of 20 **(pg 56)**
	  • Table crunches/ 4 sets of 20 **(pg 53)**
	  • Leg lifts/ 4 sets of 20 **(pg 52)**
	  • Dumbbell single leg mini crunches 3 sets of 10 (each side) **(pg 89)**

Day5 Slow jog 4 miles	**The Mix up** 1. Dumbbell flys/ 4 sets of 20 **(pg 65)** 2. Underhand dumbbell rows/ 4 sets of 20 **(pg 70)** 3. Dumbbell kickbacks / 4 sets of 20 **(pg 81)** 4. Dumbbell lunges / 4 sets of 20 **(pg 74)** 5. Flipped dumbbell shrugs/ 4 sets of 20 **(pg 85)** (Abbs) -- • Choose any 5 abdominal exercises from the book. Perform 4 sets of 20 repetitions per exercise. Be sure to switch sides for exercises that only hit one side of the abdominals at a time.
Day6 **Optional** 3-5 mile walk	**Abbs** • Choose any 5 abdominal exercises from the book. Perform 4 sets of 20 repetitions per exercise. Be sure to switch sides for exercises that only hit one side of the abdominals at a time.
Day7 **Optional** 3-5 mile walk	**Abbs** • Choose any 5 abdominal exercises from the book. Perform 4 sets of 20 repetitions per exercise. Be sure to switch sides for exercises that only hit one side of the abdominals at a time..

Week 15 Cardio	Training routine
Day1 Slow jog 4 miles	• Vertical scissors / 4 sets of 10 **(pg 55)** • Muay Thai knee/ 4 sets of 10 (each side) **(pg 59)** • Dumbbell single leg mini crunches 3 sets of 10 (each side) **(pg 89)** • Leg lifts/ 4 sets of 10 **(pg 52)** • Table crunches/ 4 sets of 10 **(pg 53)** • Plank holds/ 3 sets/ hold the plank position 3 times. Once the burn starts, count down from 20 then stop. **(pg 57)** • Extended arm to leg lifts/ 4 sets of 10 **(pg 51)** • Dumbbell chest crunches / 4 sets of 10 **(pg 88)**
Day2 Slow jog 4 miles	• Vertical scissors / 4 sets of 10 **(pg 55)** • Muay Thai knee/ 4 sets of 10 (each side) **(pg 59)** • Dumbbell single leg mini crunches 3 sets of 10 (each side) **(pg 89)** • Leg lifts/ 4 sets of 10 **(pg 52)** • Table crunches/ 4 sets of 10 **(pg 53)** • Abdominal exhales / 4 sets of 10 **(pg 60)** • Extended arm to leg lifts/ 4 sets of 10 **(pg 51)** • Dumbbell chest crunches / 4 sets of 10 **(pg 88)** • Dumbbell table crunches/ 4 sets of 10 **(pg 87)**
Day3 Slow jog 4 miles	• Vertical scissors / 4 sets of 10 **(pg 55)** • Muay Thai knee/ 4 sets of 10 (each side) **(pg 59)** • Dumbbell single leg mini crunches 3 sets of 10 (each side) **(pg 89)** • Leg lifts/ 4 sets of 10 **(pg 52)** • Table crunches/ 4 sets of 10 **(pg 53)** • Plank holds/ 3 sets/ hold the plank position 3 times. Once the burn starts, count down from 10 then stop. **(pg 57)** • Extended arm to leg lifts/ 4 sets of 10 **(pg 51)** • Dumbbell chest crunches / 4 sets of 10 **(pg 88)** • Dumbbell single leg mini crunches 3 sets of 10 (each side) **(pg 89)**

Week 15 Cardio	Training routine
Day4 Slow jog 4 miles	• Vertical scissors / 4 sets of 10 **(pg 55)** • Muay Thai knee/ 4 sets of 10 (each side) **(pg 59)** • Dumbbell single leg mini crunches 3 sets of 10 (each side) **(pg 89)** • Leg lifts/ 4 sets of 10 **(pg 52)** • Table crunches/ 4 sets of 10 **(pg 53)** • Abdominal exhales / 4 sets of 10 **(pg 60)** • Extended arm to leg lifts/ 4 sets of 10 **(pg 51)** • Dumbbell chest crunches / 4 sets of 10 **(pg 88)** • Dumbbell table crunches/ 4 sets of 10 **(pg 87)**
Day5 Slow jog 4 miles	• Vertical scissors / 3 sets of 10 **(pg 55)** • Single leg bridge lifts/ 3 sets of 10 (each side) **(pg 54)** • Parallel side scissors/ 3 sets of 10 **(pg 56)** • Leg lifts/ 3 sets of 10 **(pg 52)** • Table crunches/ 3 sets of 10 **(pg 53)** • Plank holds/ 3 sets/ hold the plank position 3 times. Once the burn starts, count down from 20 then stop. **(pg 57)** • Extended arm to leg lifts/ 3 sets of 10 **(pg 51)** • Dumbbell chest crunches / 3 sets of 10 **(pg 88)**
Day6 **Optional** 2-4 mile walk	**Abbs** • Choose any 5 abdominal exercises from the book. Perform 4 sets of 20 repetitions per exercise. Be sure to switch sides for exercises that only hit one side of the abdominals at a time.
Day7 **Optional** 2-4 mile walk	**Abbs** • Choose any 5 abdominal exercises from the book. Perform 4 sets of 20 repetitions per exercise. Be sure to switch sides for exercises that only hit one side of the abdominals at a time.

Week 16 Cardio	Training routine
Day1 Slow jog 5 miles	1. <u>Dumbbell lateral raises/ 10 sets of 20</u> **(pg 82)** • Vertical scissors / 4 sets of 10 **(pg 55)** • Muay Thai knee/ 4 sets of 10 (each side) **(pg 59)** • Dumbbell single leg mini crunches 3 sets of 10 (each side) **(pg 89)** • Leg lifts/ 4 sets of 10 **(pg 52)** • Table crunches/ 4 sets of 10 **(pg 53)** • Plank Holds/ 3 sets/ hold the plank position 3 times. Once the burn starts, count down from 30 then stop. **(pg 57)** • Extended arm to leg lifts/ 4 sets of 10 **(pg 51)** • Dumbbell chest crunches / 4 sets of 10 **(pg 88)**
Day2 Slow jog 5 miles	1. <u>Dumbbell turns/ 10 sets of 20</u> **(pg 66)** • Vertical scissors / 4 sets of 10 **(pg 55)** • Muay Thai knee/ 4 sets of 10 (each side) **(pg 59)** • Dumbbell single leg mini crunches 3 sets of 10 (each side) **(pg 89)** • Leg lifts/ 4 sets of 10 **(pg 52)** • Table crunches/ 4 sets of 10 **(pg 53)** • Abdominal exhales / 4 sets of 10 **(pg 60)** • Extended arm to leg lifts/ 4 sets of 10 **(pg 51)** • Dumbbell chest crunches / 4 sets of 10 **(pg 88)** • Dumbbell table crunches/ 4 sets of 10 **(pg 87)**
Day3 Slow jog 5 miles	1. <u>Dumbbell curls/ 10 sets of 20</u> **(pg 79)** • Vertical scissors / 4 sets of 10 **(pg 55)** • Muay Thai knee/ 4 sets of 10 (each side) **(pg 59)** • Dumbbell single leg mini crunches 3 sets of 10 (each side) **(pg 89)** • Leg lifts/ 4 sets of 10 **(pg 52)** • Table crunches/ 4 sets of 10 **(pg 53)** • Plank Holds/ 3 sets/ hold the plank position 3 times. Once the burn starts, count down from 10 then stop. **(pg 57)** • Extended arm to leg lifts/ 4 sets of 10 **(pg 51)** • Dumbbell chest crunches / 4 sets of 10 **(pg 88)**

Week 16 Cardio	Training routine
Day4 Slow jog 5 miles	1. <u>Parallel dumbbell squats/ 10 sets of 20</u> **(pg 75)** • Vertical scissors / 4 sets of 10 **(pg 55)** • Muay Thai knee/ 4 sets of 10 (each side) **(pg 59)** • Dumbbell single leg mini crunches 3 sets of 10 (each side) **(pg 89)** • Leg lifts/ 4 sets of 10 **(pg 52)** • Table crunches/ 4 sets of 10 **(pg 53)** • Abdominal exhales / 4 sets of 10 **(pg 60)** • Extended arm to leg lifts/ 4 sets of 10 **(pg 51)** • Dumbbell chest crunches / 4 sets of 10 **(pg 88)** • Dumbbell table crunches/ 4 sets of 10 **(pg 87)**
Day5 Slow jog 5 miles	1. <u>Dumbbell deadlifts / 8 sets of 20</u> **(pg 72)** • Vertical scissors / 3 sets of 10 **(pg 55)** • Single leg bridge lifts/ 3 sets of 10 (each side) **(pg 54)** • Parallel side scissors/ 3 sets of 10 **(pg 56)** • Leg lifts/ 3 sets of 10 **(pg 52)** • Table crunches/ 3 sets of 10 **(pg 53)** • Plank holds/ 3 sets/ hold the plank position 3 times. Once the burn starts, count down from 10 then stop. **(pg 57)** • Extended arm to leg lifts/ 3 sets of 10 **(pg 51)** • Dumbbell chest crunches / 3 sets of 10 **(pg 88)**
Day6 **Optional** 2-4 mile walk	**Abbs** • Choose any 5 abdominal exercises from the book. Perform 4 sets of 20 repetitions per exercise. Be sure to switch sides for exercises that only hit one side of the abdominals at a time.
Day7 **Optional** 2-4 mile walk	**Abbs** • Choose any 5 abdominal exercises from the book. Perform 4 sets of 20 repetitions per exercise. Be sure to switch sides for exercises that only hit one side of the abdominals at a time.

If by (week/step) 16 you do not have your Hollywood abbs out, alternate between weeks 12, 14, 15 and 16. Keep doing this until you achieve the results you are striving for. If you don't eat crap food, getting those abbs will be a hell of a lot faster.

(Note) Once you achieve your Hollywood abbs objective, be sure to keep up the maintenance work. Mixing up weeks (8-15) in any order is recommended as an ongoing maintenance routine; if you do not implement other forms of training.

CHAPTER 9
THE HOLLYWOOD ABBS FOOD LIST

Hollywood abbs without a clean diet is something unheard of. If you cannot eat clean, you might still get lean by following the 16 week training plan, but getting lean and getting those Hollywood abbs out are two different things. Getting lean simply means looking better than the average persona. Getting the Hollywood abbs out means getting ripped.

Something to consider <u>if you are on a tight abbs schedule with a deadline</u>

1) Forget about counting calories.
2) Forget about dairy products 95 percent of the time.
3) Forget that candy, junk food and sugary drinks exist.
4) If you have the opportunity to talk to a bodybuilder who competed in <u>multiple</u> shows, he or she may provide you with additional expert dieting information.
   (Note) The 16 week training approach is different from that of what a bodybuilder takes before a contest, but the diet is very similar.
5) Most of the time it's the food that trips people up, not the training. (Remember the Hollywood abbs commandment #1).
6) If you drop the carbs too low, you will experience low blood sugar and other possible negative psychological/ physical side effects. Be sure to carb up every morning.
7) Most nutritionist will not agree with the overall dietary approach. Remember, what you are doing is (level 3 - 4 training). This is the level of intensity (food and training) many stars go through to get those abbs out. You can even think of the food in this chapter as the 11th commandment. "11th commandment (If the food items you think of are not on this chapters list, it's a good possibility that the excluded items are less effective)."

(Note) Many other healthy foods are available. But, you are thinking ripped abbs as priority. <u>Not all healthy foods impact the image sculpting part of the equation equally.</u> Eating healthy food and eating food that can help you get those abbs out are not entirely the same. All though most healthy foods from this chapter's list may overlap with general healthy foods, there is a constraint to options. In no way are you being told that you should not eat other healthy foods, however chomping down on bananas, grapes and yogurt all day will not help. Is it healthy? Yes. Will it help you get those abbs out? Not really.

8) Don't forget that once a week you could go out and have a cheat meal. A cheat meal is not to be confused with a cheat day. (Hollywood abbs commandment #5).

9) It might not be a bad idea to throw in fish oil and a multi vitamin into the mix.

10) For those who choose to include fat burners and caffeine in the overall routine, take at least one or two days off from stimulants every week. These things are not the healthiest things in the world, but because many will still use them regardless of what I say, keep in mind that you have been warned. Stimulant dependency may occur if you do not regularly take brakes.

The Hollywood abbs food list

Protein--

Skinless chicken breasts-(grilled)(baked)(broiled)(boiled)
If someone asked what's the ultimate Hollywood abbs protein. The answer would be chicken. Skinless chicken breasts to be exact.

- Low on calories
- High protein
- Low fat
- No sugar
- No carbs
- Filling

Fish- isn't just a good source of protein, it's also an exellent source of omage-3 fatty acids. The omega-3's have numerous health benefits. When someone is in hard training, eating fish is highly recommended.

- Good source of protein
- Good source of healthy fats
- No sugar
- No carbs
- Filling

- Easy on digestion

Turkey meat or ground turkey

Not all turkey products are cratered equal. To get those Hollywood abbs, do not eat the prepackaged deli turkey products. They are loaded with sodium. Try to buy the lean 93%, 97% or 99% fat free ground turkey meat. Ground turkey cooked up with a little olive oil and bell peppers topped off with a low sodium seasoning serves as an excellent dinner choice.

- Good source of protein
- No sugar
- No carbs
- Usually sold at a good price

Egg whites

When in doubt what to eat after a workout, go for the egg whites. The low calorie, high protein egg white meal is absorbed faster than meat and takes minutes to make. Pour some egg whites from a prepackaged egg white carton on to a hot pan and you are almost done. The egg white omelet is a fabulous idea for someone who has little time to eat or cook.

- Fast
- Easy
- Low on calories
- No sugar
- No carbs
- Good source of protein
- Protein is absorbed fast
- Easy on digestion

Top sirloin lean steak

Because red meat is high in cholesterol, it's not a good idea to make a habit of eating steak all the time. However, a lean steak is high in protein, and it does help eating steak once in a while with some vegetables to get those Hollywood abbs out from underneath the fat. Go easy on the seasoning and the steak sauce. Instead of sauce or seasoning, try substituting with fresh lightly salted salsa.

- No sugar
- No carbs
- Good source of protein
- Filling

Plain tofu- Is considered to be a healthy weight loss food by many. By itself, tofu may be bland so mix it up with something to add flavor.

- Low or no cholesterol
- Low sodium
- Good source of protein
- No sugar
- No carbs
- Easy on digestion
- Low on calories

The protein shake-All though a protein shake is not to be considered as food, but as a supplement, it earns the right to be on the list. A standard protein shake should never replace a meal, that's a fact. However, on numerous occasions there is no time to eat. A post workout protein shake is always a good idea.

- Good source of protein
- Fast absorption
- Low on calories
- Portable

Energy /Carbs--

Plain instant oatmeal- Perhaps the best way to start the day right is with a bowl of plain instant oatmeal and some fruit. Oatmeal is a good source of fiber and complex carbohydrates.
- Good source of complex carbohydrates
- Good source of fiber
- Filling
- Source of protein
- Helps with digestion

Rice cakes
This low calorie carbohydrate snack is packed with whole grain nutrients and cuts massive amounts of calories from the diet. The hard core Hollywood abbs individuals prefer the salt free Quaker rice cakes.

- Low on calories
- Portable
- Low or no fat
- Low or no sodium

Brown rice (steamed)

Steamed brown rice is similar in relation to oatmeal. It's a good source of fiber and complex carbohydrates. Be careful, it's easy to misjudge portion size and eat too much rice in one sitting. Have brown rice as a side to a main course meat meal. Try to have twice the amount of vegetables on the plate in ratio to rice.

- Good source of complex carbohydrates
- Good source of fiber
- Filling

Buckwheat (steamed)(boiled)

Buckwheat aka "strong man food" is not found in all stores, but it is well worth the search.

- Good source of complex carbohydrates
- Good source of fiber
- Filling
- Low or no fat
- No sodium
- Source of protein

Small apples

Small apples are a good source of fiber and natural sugar. Whenever a feeling of weakness comes over and you just flat out hit the wall, besides the protein shake, a rush of natural sugar from a small apple is a good idea.

- Low on calories
- No fat
- Quick natural energy (natural sugar)

Small baked potatoes (plain)

A plain baked potato can be one of your best friends. A loaded fancy baked potato can be one of your worst enemies. A baked potato goes well with; fish, meat, chicken and turkey. Besides being a good source of quality complex carbohydrates, it's also a source of vitamin C.

- Good source of complex carbohydrates
- Filling
- Low or no fat

Yam (plain baked)

Yams are an amazing source of complex carbohydrates that taste like cake when baked in the oven. When someone is following a strict diet for a long time, this tasty side dish just may satisfy a sweet tooth. Nothing like some steamed broccoli with fish and a small baked yam.

- Good source of complex carbohydrates
- Filling
- Low or no fat

Good fats--

Avocados

Avocados contain good fat. Throw in some avocados into the diet.

- Good fats (monounsaturated fats)
- Natural antioxidants
- Heart health

Plain almonds

As healthy as almonds are, they are highly caloric. Eat them sparingly or mix them into salads.
- Good fats (monounsaturated fats)
- Heart health
- Source of protein

Extra virgin olive oil

When cooking chicken or steak on the open flame it's a good idea to lightly code the meat with extra virgin olive oil. This will allow the meat to stay juicy. If you never used olive oil on chicken or meat I'm sure that sometimes the final product came out dry. Lightly coding the meat with olive oil solves that problem.

- Good fats (monounsaturated fats)
- Heart health
- Enhances flavor of meat when cooking on an open flame

Fish (mentioned earlier)
Plain tofu products (mentioned earlier)

The Hollywood abbs antioxidants /vitamins --

Mixed leafy greens
Spinach
Avocado (mentioned earlier)
Lettuce
Tomatoes
Cucumbers
Broccoli
Asparagus
Bell peppers
Onions
Lemons
Limes
Garlic
Green onion
Brussels sprouts

Other Important Hollywood abbs food elements-------------------------------------

Water
Stay hydrated when training. (Always).

Example

Current weight   200
Divide by   2
Amount of oz   100

The person who weighs 200lbs and trains on a daily basis should drink 100 oz of water per day as a general guideline.

1 gallon = 128.00oz
1 liter =   33.81 oz
Standard water bottle 16oz

Low sodium seasoning

Excessive sodium in the diet leads to additional water retention. If you are holding on to excessive water weight, when you drop the fat, your Hollywood abbs will be flat. Low sodium seasoning adds the flavor without the salt.

(Note) Please DO NOT get diuretics and water pills. Simply be patient, drink lots of water and use low sodium seasoning.

(Warning) While training hard, misuse of diuretics and water pills can land the person into a hospital or worse.

Mustard

Plain mustard has zero calories.

Fresh blueberries

Can be eaten with oatmeal to enhance the overall taste. A good snack.

- Low on calories
- No fat
- Quick natural energy (natural sugar)
- Source of fiber

Fresh strawberries

Can be eaten with oatmeal to enhance the overall taste. A good snack.

- Low on calories
- No fat
- Quick natural energy (natural sugar)
- Source of fiber

CHAPTER 10
THE 555 METHOD

The 555 method is perhaps one of the most effective approaches to consider when attempting to drop body fat and getting those Hollywood abbs out. This simple, effective training approach can do wonders in the overall image modification department.

This method was specifically included in this book because a large percentage of individuals prefer to only train in a gym setting. This method may be applied in the gym as well as outside the gym.

A few things to consider

1. It takes time to work up to this training method.

2. All weight bearing exercises must be executed thoroughly.

3. Rushing through this type of training without control opens a wider possibility to injury.

4. Always warm up before training (especially when applying the 555 method).

5. Always stretch after the warm up.

6. The Hollywood abbs commandments apply.

7. The Hollywood abbs foods apply.

8. Do not use heavy weight.

9. Because you will be sculpting your body and burning calories like crazy, be sure to carb up for breakfast. (Always).

10. It is possible that you may not be in top condition to apply this method of training five days a week. As time progresses, work up to using the 555 method for most training days of the week.

The 555 Method

- **500 reps per major body part trained in one session through multiple exercises.**

- **50 minutes of intensive cardiovascular training after working out the major body part.**

- **5 small clean meals per day.**

   500 reps + 50 minutes intense cardio + 5 clean meals = 555

The sequence of training in the example below does not have to be executed in the presented format.

Example

Monday- Chest- 500 reps (abbs optional 100 reps)+(50 min cardio)+(5 clean meals)

Tuesday- Back- 500 reps (abbs optional 100 reps)+(50 min cardio)+(5 clean meals)

Wednesday- Legs 500 reps (abbs optional 100 reps)+(50 min cardio)+(5 clean meals)

Thursday- OFF (or) (Abbs training 500 reps)+(50 min cardio)+(5 clean meals)

Friday- Arms 500 reps (abbs optional 100 reps)+(50 min cardio)+(5 clean meals)

Saturday- Shoulders 500 reps (abbs optional 100 reps)+(50 min cardio)+(5 clean meals)

Sunday- OFF (or) (Abbs training 500 reps)+(50 min cardio)+(5 clean meals)

Additional notes on the 555 method

- A Protein shake does not count as a meal, but it is a must after the training session.

- If you are not showered in sweat after the 50 minutes of cardio, the cardio was not intense enough.

- You might be tempted to throw in another body part to complete the daily 500 repetitions. Example (250 reps for the chest and 250 reps for the back). Do not do that. Stop where you are. Take note of how many repetitions you did for the body part you are training and attempt to beat that rep number the following week. Keep doing this till you can comfortably do 500 reps per body part/ per workout.

"I wish you good luck on any and all positive goals you set out to achieve in life. Keep moving forward and most of all, believe in yourself."

Thank you
Ilya

Ilya Sulima

ANOTHER BOOK BY ILYA SULIMA
"RUSSIAN RIPPED"

ПРАВДА

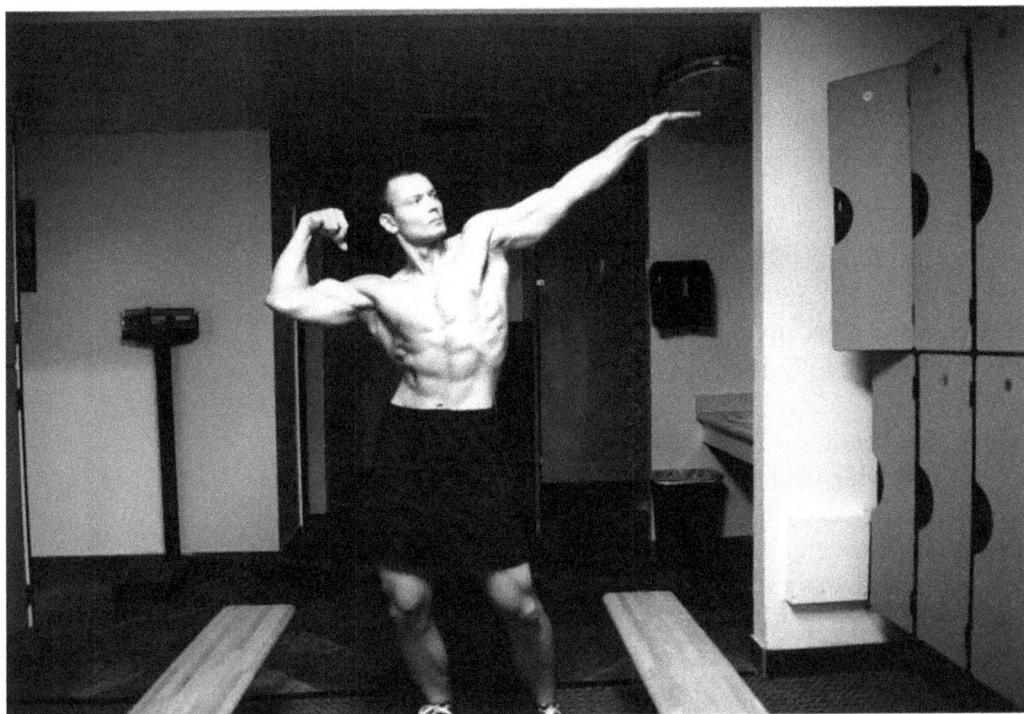

RUSSIAN RIPPED
THE COLD WAR IS OVER
GET RIPPED THE RUSSIAN WAY

ILYA SULIMA

www.Ilyasulima.com

Shortened Reference Index

www.ingramcontent.com/pod-product-compliance
Lightning Source LLC
Chambersburg PA
CBHW081416270326
41931CB00015B/3294